A History of Rhetoric, Sound, and Health and Healing

A History of Rhetoric, Sound, and Health and Healing argues for medico-sonic knowledge—systematically interpreted bodily sounds with medical knowledge mediated by rhetoric—as an evolving corporeal practice with an incomparable, sprawling history.

Taking a materialist-feminist perspective, the book rhetorically accounts for sound and suggests rhetoric enables bodily sounds as understandable, knowable, and treatable with power to help and discipline bodies in health, healing, and hospital contexts. From an expansive, pan-historiographic approach integrated with and influenced by fieldwork from neonatal intensive care units (NICUs) in Denmark and the United States, the author explores intentional and unintentional diagnostic, prognostic, and therapeutic uses of sound in contemporary Western biomedical health systems and promotes a new research concept and fieldwork practice, sound in all research.

The insightful, timely volume will interest students and researchers in the medical humanities, rhetoric and communication, health communication, sound studies, medical and allied health sciences, and research methods.

Kristin Marie Bivens is a scholar of the Rhetoric of Health and Medicine and the head of education in the Department of Clinical Research at the University of Bern in Switzerland. She also heads the patient and public involvement program in clinical research.

Routledge Studies in Rhetoric and Communication

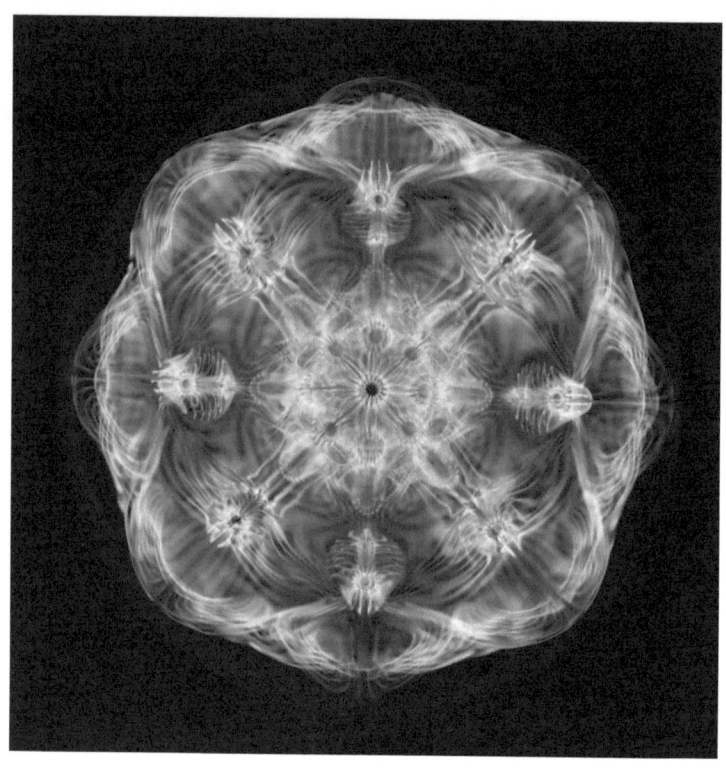

Linden Gledhill. *Cymatics, standing sound waves.* Photograph. 2016. Used with permission. https://www.flickr.com/photos/13084997@N03/24654244819/in/album-72157664382425281/

A History of Rhetoric, Sound, and Health and Healing

Kristin Marie Bivens

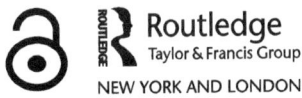

Routledge
Taylor & Francis Group
NEW YORK AND LONDON

First published 2025
by Routledge
605 Third Avenue, New York, NY 10158

and by Routledge
4 Park Square, Milton Park, Abingdon, Oxon, OX14 4RN

Routledge is an imprint of the Taylor & Francis Group, an informa business

© 2025 Kristin Marie Bivens

Library of Congress Cataloging-in-Publication Data
Names: Bivens, Kristin Marie, author.
Title: A history of rhetoric, sound, and health and healing / Kristin Marie Bivens.
Description: New York, NY : Routledge, 2025. |
Series: Routledge studies in rhetoric and communication |
Includes bibliographical references and index.
Identifiers: LCCN 2024030866 (print) | LCCN 2024030867 (ebook) |
ISBN 9781032724379 (hardback) | ISBN 9781032724409 (paperback) |
ISBN 9781032724416 (ebook)
Subjects: LCSH: Sound--Therapeutic use. | Communication in medicine. |
Feminism and rhetoric. | Medicine and the humanities. |
Medical anthropology.
Classification: LCC R130 .B528 2025 (print) |
LCC R130 (ebook) | DDC 616.001/4--dc23/eng/20240820
LC record available at https://lccn.loc.gov/2024030866
LC ebook record available at https://lccn.loc.gov/2024030867

ISBN: 978-1-032-72437-9 (hbk)
ISBN: 978-1-032-72440-9 (pbk)
ISBN: 978-1-032-72441-6 (ebk)

DOI: 10.4324/9781032724416

Typeset in Times New Roman
by KnowledgeWorks Global Ltd.

Access the Support Material: //www.routledge.com/9781032724379

To Gustav, Lou, and Fifi. And to farmor.

Contents

Acknowledgments

My bountiful appreciation is dedicated to a series of people—wonderful, influential, and otherwise—who offered their support, guidance, and contrast throughout the writing of *A History of Rhetoric, Sound, and Health and Healing* from its formative stage as a journal article in the *Rhetoric of Health of Medicine* to its now publication as monograph.

The idea for focusing on sound in health and healing emanates from a question Kelli Cargile Cook (KCC) asked me at the very, very end of my PhD defense nearly a decade ago about my multisite, multicountry study: what do neonatal intensive care units (NICUs) in Copenhagen, Denmark, and Texas have in common? The only item I could reasonably state were physiological monitors. The question and my response prompted later examining the sounds of a NICU more closely and intentionally.

To the City Colleges of Chicago and Harold Washington College for a sabbatical leave to research and learn about Denmark in Denmark. I am especially appreciative of Local 1600 for their unending commitment to creating the best working conditions and benefits for faculty—my research sabbatical continues as an unparalleled perk of my career to date. To my former colleagues in the English department, thank you. I am also grateful for financial support from the Helen Locke Carter Memorial Grant Research fund from Texas Tech University (TTU). To my PhD cohort—the Infin8s—at TTU (and all the other cohort members), thank you. I also found a vibrant intellectual space as a Newberry Library Scholar-in-Residence in Chicago and inspiration for which I offer my appreciation.

To the nurses, parents, and carers of premature and sick infants at the Rigshospitalet in Copenhagen, Denmark, and in the United States who participated in my study, thank you for trusting me during such a time in your life. I offer my specific appreciation to the NICU at St. John's Hospital (SJH) in Springfield, Illinois—I became curious about communication from experiences in the NICU at SJH. I thank Alyce Ashcraft and Pam Lackey from Texas Tech University Health Science Center and University Medical Center, as well as Janne Weiss and Ragnhild Maastrup from the Rigshospitalet Neonatalklinnikken in Copenhagen, Denmark.

The Rhetoric of Health and Medicine (RHM) crew is a spicy gang of savvy scholars who helped shape my research and work since my first symposium in Cincinnati in 2015 with a mix of laughter, libations, and kindness. Catherine Gouge, Blake Scott, Molly Kessler, Amy Koerber (more appreciation for her soon), Jennifer Malkowski, Carie S. Tucker King, Debra Burleson, Lisa Melonçon, Lora Arduser, Liz Angeli, Candice A. Welhausen (CAW), Laura Pigozzi, and all those who participated in RHM activities, such as the goblet of inquiry.

To the incomparable Sherena Huntsman for encouragement and entertaining my questions about her chickens (and so much more). Tim J. Elliot: thanks for your friendship and openness to wax technical communication whenever (and thank you for the opportunity to speak about my research to your department at DePaul University). To CAW—our albatross made the monograph seem easy in comparison. Kirsti Cole—my first scholar-friend, my first co-author, and the best feminist. Amy Koerber, thank you for working with me all these years and answering my very first email to you so quickly in 2011—I have felt your support and friendship since; from the Rocky Mountain Writer's Retreat to the Alsace Writer's Retreat, thank you.

Like others, the pandemic effortlessly split my life into a before and an after. I began writing the pages of the book during a two-month stopover in Sweden before moving to Switzerland in summer 2020. Although our intention was to return to Chicago after one year, we found our way in Bern, Switzerland—the country with the sweetest spring-smelling air and the sweetest carrots.

At the University of Bern's Institute of Social and Preventive Medicine (ISPM), I thank Chris Ritter, Beatrice Minder, and Doris Kopp (and the whole Zentrale Dienste crew) for easy conversations about books and sharing knowledge for finding information I sought. I also thank the authors I worked with at ISPM as the scientific editor—your work influenced me in ways I'm still realizing.

A special thanks to the students at the University of Bern in the Public Health Science's Qualitative Research Living Lab II (2023–2024) who motivated me to remember to rest in many ways and write when inspired.

I also appreciate support and conversations with my colleagues in the Department of Clinical Research at the University of Bern—it's a dynamic place dripping with opportunities and bright intellects. Thank you—Eva Segelov—for bringing me over and introducing me to such opportunities.

A History of Rhetoric, Sound, and Health and Healing is published—as gold open access—with the support of the Swiss National Science Foundation for scientific research. The pre-press stage of this publication was also supported by the Swiss National Science Foundation for scientific research.

A sincere thank you to Suzanne Richardson and Stuti Goel from Routledge and the external manuscript reviewers, as well as everyone who worked on publishing this work. Thank you. I also thank Allie Boman for her editorial work and guidance on what eventually became chapters 2 and 3 and also her team's work on the index.

A dear friend and her children gave me a yellow stethoscope as a gift at a party we hosted in Chicago to celebrate passing my PhD defense—I keep it hanging nearby my home office workspace in Switzerland. VP explained the gift from her children. She said it's because I was now a doctor, so I needed a stethoscope. I remember thinking such a gift was thoughtful and cute, yet now I know it as something else, something more of a beacon or harbinger.

To my oldest, dearest friend—the one who knows, knows it all—Jamie. When we were children, your zest and commitment for reading sparked something within me that shines brightly today. You shared your books with me; it was the ultimate act of kindness and friendship.

For over a decade, my darling partner, Gustav, has supported my writing (even now as I write this, and he offers to take the dog out for her Sunday evening walk so I can continue writing). It's been a wild ride, so far; I look forward to more of it, s.p.

And I thank you, kind reader, for understanding how intentions of accuracy and interpretation do not always result in accurate interpretations— I tried to get it right; I hope I did. It is a pan-historiography, not a history.

1 Sound and Rhetoric in Health and Healing

A Conflux of Rhetoric and Sound

Written, spoken, and visual[i] language does much for making sense of the world and sharing our experiences; sound does, too. Without a millennia-long interplay between rhetoric and sound, *science-based, allopathic Western biomedicine*—the predominant medical system that treats symptoms and diseases with drugs, interventions, and operations—would not exist as we know it. With rhetoric, the body's sounds are understandable, knowable, and treatable. My working definition of sound is rhetorically oriented, materialist-feminist, and meaning-giving; it expands upon Joshua Gunn, Greg Goodale, Mirko M. Hall, and Rosa A. Eberly's definition: "vibrations in the air [or water] that can be heard or felt by most [hearing] animals,"[1] emanating from and potentially impacting nonhuman objects, as well. It also draws from Dominic Pettman when he attends to hearing abilities by adding "vibrations are the interface between the experience of an ear that functions as designed and one that does not, since no one—not even the profoundly deaf—can escape the sonic 'feeling' of sound waves,"[2] which is also evident in the Linden Gledhill cymatic image of sound displayed opposite the title page. Yet, I further distinguish between those vibrations and the sound—as either purposeful or unintentional—a departure from Richard Marback's contention in rhetorical studies that "Giving objects their due … requires of us that we do attend to what gets done without appeal to an intentionality or a representation that overdetermines what ought to be done."[3]

My distinction is especially attuned to vibration and sound or noise in *health, healing, and hospital contexts*—places where approaches, interventions, or treatments are used to enhance, recover, and repair toward an ideal bodily human experience—where the body's sounds are amplified through healthcare technologies, such as stethoscopes or physiological monitors, and when unchecked or only mildly regulated, scatter like sonic shrapnel in environments where they are heard and felt. For example, a health context might include a yoga class; a healing context, an acupuncture session with a Chinese medicine practitioner; and a hospital context, a medical surgical ward

---

i I specifically mean sign language.

DOI: 10.4324/9781032724416-1

for post-operative hospitalized individuals. Yet, health, healing, and hospital contexts are interrelated, as well, since all concern approaches, interventions, or treatments used to enhance, recover, and repair—or improve—the quality of our lives. Health, healing, and hospital represent different contexts where people seek relief and general assistance feeling better.

I contend sound and its rhetorical power are often overlooked, as well as its role helping, healing, and harming in health, healing, and hospital contexts. Molly Kessler writes, "We must rhetorically and reflectively listen if we want to ethically engage with each other's lived experiences, particularly in the contexts of health and medicine."[4] She identifies Annemarie Mol's praxiography or "ethnography of practices"[5] "as a way to understand the rhetorical work in peoples' lived experiences."[6] Scholars of the rhetoric of health and medicine (RHM)—as Kessler points out[7]—have used praxiography in an array of discursive contexts. The underlying assumption of praxiography is attention to "theories and approaches that encourage us to focus on the perspectives, perceptions, interpretations, even descriptions of a singular, stable reality."[8] In my estimation, "listening" is a stand in for such praxiographic attention—it does not mean hearing necessarily. Instead, it is rhetorical shorthand for giving attention or drawing attention to what counts, what is worthy of noting or amplifying—it is materialist-feminist.

Feminism is about drawing attention to what counts, what is worthy of noting or amplifying. The underlying assumption informing my examination of sound in health in healing is that it is valuable. Sound in health and healing can be intentional and helpful, providing diagnostic, prognostic, and therapeutic possibilities, while noise is unintentional and potentially disruptive, yet also revelatory. Whether in the air or water, vibratory effects from nonhuman actors, such as healthcare technologies, shape action. When vibrations gather, the energy they produce causes sound. Sound is simply vibration, yet when vibrations assemble, they can be powerful sonic forces that spur action, require attention, and shape experiences for hearing and deaf bodies alike. To illustrate in a hospital context, TikTok creator @nurse_sushi[9] comments on an omnipresent or "continuous wave"[10] of ICU physiological alarms for the unit's 30 patients with COVID-19 infections. @nurse_sushi points out in the video's accompanying caption: "Alarm fatigue is high these days." *Alarm fatigue*[11] occurs when nurses are "exposed to an excessive number of alarms, which can result in desensitization to alarms and missed alarms."[12] Deciphering or translating what sounds from healthcare technologies indicate requires specialist knowledge often gained from a combination of formal training and clinical experience. Implying viewers possibly do not possess such *medico-sonic knowledge*—bodily sounds systematically interpreted through medical knowledge mediated by rhetoric— @nurse_sushi's textual narration starts the video by asking viewers and listeners,

Did you guys know that COVID has a sound? Once the patient is intubated and sedated, which is all 30 of our ICU beds right now. You think that the patients can't make any kind of noise. They just make different kinds of noise right now.

In the rest of the video, she provides about 70 seconds of written commentary; the audio that punctuates the remainder of the video features the nonstop sounds of ventilators alarming to indicate breathing or difficulties related to bodily vital functions. @nurse_sushi offers written commentary in the video: "These are red alarms, they are the loudest alarm and mean a vital sign has reached a critical limit...."

Healthcare technologies, such as physiological monitors and ventilators, amplify the body's heart, lung, and intestinal sounds, then those sounds are interpreted by trained healthcare clinicians, such as nurses or physicians, who give medico-sonic meaning to the body's sounds. In the example of @nurse_sushi, the intentional effect from amplifying the body's sounds is present in her expert interpretation of them; she states, "a vital sign has reached a critical limit." However, the unintentional effect she references is alarm fatigue. When unchecked or only mildly regulated, healthcare technology sounds have resulted in alarm fatigue. Although physiological monitors and other healthcare technologies provide meaningful and purposeful sounds to alert clinicians and provide life-saving care, alarm fatigue has been associated with negatively impacting patient care,[13] causing patient deaths,[14,15] and, anecdotally, stressing out @nurse_sushi. Sound, the body, and its environment are inseparable; @nurse_sushi highlights "the often unpredictable and unwanted actions of human bodies"[16] that Stacy Alaimo describes by referencing her alarm fatigue—a phenomenon hearing bodies experience because we do not have "earlids,"[17] yet impact all bodies, whether hearing or deaf.

Later in @nurse_sushi's video, she continues her textual narration while the alarms continue to sound unpleasantly; she remarks, "This is what we hear all night, because we can't drop [adjust] the alarm parameters anymore ...," then adds "Your nurses are literally listening to you starve for oxygen knowing there is nothing more we can do." Before reminding viewers to get vaccinated, she claims, "Soon, your heart, tired of oxygen starvation, will arrest." @nurse_sushi describes the clinical term hypoxia as oxygen starvation, using rhetorical personification to do so. @nurse_sushi's use of rhetoric is meaningful, yet unoriginal. As I argue throughout *A History of Rhetoric, Sound, and Health and Healing*, the use of rhetorical devices to describe and make sense of our bodies are legacies of health and healing from ancient civilizations in Mesopotamia, Egypt, India, Greece, and Italy (and likely elsewhere). Although the stethoscope inventor and French physician René Theophile-Hyacinthe Laënnec popularized auscultating (or listening to) the heart, lungs, and other organs, as well as provided a textbook for gathering medico-sonic interpretations of the body, throughout known recorded history sound has signaled bodily health used to promote healing.

In many ways, this book is about using rhetoric to make meaning with the sonic qualities of our bodies and from making our bodies sonic. Yet, it is also about how sound is used to signal health and vitality. For example, consider Hansen's disease or leprosy. In Europe during the Middle Ages, bells were reportedly used to announce the approach of people with leprosy (who wore clothing that alerted uninfected others that they had the disease).[18] In medieval Europe, it was also thought that people infected with leprosy used bells and wooden clappers to announce their presence.[19] However, some historians have used medieval paintings to theorize that this was not the case, instead arguing that the bells and wooden clappers were used to alert—not scare or alarm—nearby people and call for mercy.[20] Whether used to alarm or alert bystanders, as a non-discursive notification about the body's condition, sound was relied upon to sonically signal leprosy and prompt action from listeners.

Sound and Somatic Consequence

A major premise of this book derives from sound's multiple ontologies: its simultaneous, unambiguous value as an auditory beacon for communication and human listening pleasure, and its underexplored value as an influential, non-discursive source of information and connection. In health, healing, and hospital contexts, sound can be both from and directed at bodies. Whether in nature, in our bodies, or in hospital rooms, vibration as noise or sound prompts natural or biological action, often with sensory-derived somatic consequences. In my field research in a neonatal intensive care unit (NICU) in the southwestern United States, as well as in Copenhagen, Denmark, I witnessed amplified bodily sounds from infants direct attention toward a secondary source of the sound—physiological monitors—and I witnessed sound from a physiological monitor shape action beyond eye movement and noted how those sounds can be harmful:

a new father sat behind a drawn curtain with the mother and their new baby. The mother, as I observed and heard, wanted privacy while she breastfed their new baby. Since mom was not yet discharged from the hospital, she was connected to an intravenous fluid (IV) pump, which is common for [people] who have recently delivered babies. Suddenly, an alarm sounded from behind the curtain: a sharp ding–pause, ding–pause, ding–pause filled the pod from behind the closed curtain.

Not immediately, but after several minutes, the naturally concerned father responded to the alarm. Dad opened the curtain and asked me to find his baby's nurse (a man). I immediately jumped up, found his baby's nurse, and told him to come to the pod (he was helping another nurse in a different pod).

The father spoke quickly to his baby's nurse and asked for a woman nurse (since his wife was breastfeeding and presumably had exposed breasts). The baby's nurse located a woman nurse to attend to the IV pump's alarm—the reason for the father's concern.

Behind the closed (not soundproof) curtain that didn't reach the floor, the woman nurse explained that it was only the IV pump alerting to indicate mom's IV fluid bag would be empty soon—not an emergency that needed immediate attention—and the sound stopped. The woman nurse opened the curtain and exited. Within ten minutes, the alarm for the IV pump was sounding again. This time, after loudly complaining about the alarm to the mother, the father moved quickly to go find a nurse, causing him to trip and fall on the ground (as I witnessed through the gap between the curtain and floor).[21]

Discouraging direct and primary attention on patient bodies, healthcare technologies encourage initial attention to themselves and their medico-sonic representations of internal physiological functions. In this way, healthcare technologies perform an act of ventriloquism. François Cooren theorized *rhetorical ventriloquism* as a kind of "vocal artifice"[22] and a communicative element that calls upon entities and even institutions to do another's vocal bidding.[23] Cooren defined it as "the various ways by which human interactants make certain entities (collectives, procedures, policies, ideologies, etc.) speak in their name and vice versa."[24] Along with Laënnec's rhetorical devices and foundational medico-sonic understandings of the body explored in Chapter 3, rhetorical ventriloquism draws power from and reinforces science-based, allopathic Western biomedicine sometimes with punishing effects.

Nearby sounds—bodily or otherwise—and noises influence and shape our actions. Alaimo contends the material turn in feminist theory led by such theorists as Donna Haraway, Vicki Kirby, Elizabeth Wilson, and Karen Barad asks "how nonhuman nature or the human body can 'talk back,' resist, or otherwise affect its cultural construction."[25] As an example, powerful vibrations from explosions can trigger snow avalanches to release[26]; or in an ocean, underwater sonar testing can cause large hearing marine mammals to flee the water to escape sonically distressing environments.[27] Although these are somewhat extreme examples, they exemplify sound's power in the wild. In each example, nature talks back by releasing an avalanche or beaching itself, which are clearly acts of responding to and resisting sound—the somatic consequences of sound. As another extreme and injurious use of sound, consider sound's role in violence and torture. Juliane Brauer responded to a question that musicologists asked, "Can music be considered a form of torture?"[28] She chose to use examples from written accounts of life during World War II in Auschwitz-Birkenau to make her argument that

> Music was combined in Nazi concentration and extermination camps with other forms of physical and emotional torture in ways previously unimagined and to a completely new extent. In this combination music had the potential to destroy prisoners' humanity in ways that would not be possible using physical forms of torture alone.[29]

Brauer draws from scholarly and first-hand accounts to make claims about how music was used as torture in concentration and extermination camps, noting that the scholarly attention since the 1970s has resulted in "The wealth of information now available in archival and public collections allows for a reconsideration of the role of music as an instrument of torture."[30] Using the interplay of music, emotion, violence, and the body, Brauer makes a compelling historical case for the power of music as it violently and heinously interacted with the bodies and feelings of those imprisoned at these camps—the somatic consequences of sound.

All around us, we can earwitness[31] the power of sound. Yet, we have yet to comprehensively offer an account for sound's role in health, healing, and hospital contexts—how we have used non-discursive sound to make meaning from, sense of, and treatments for our bodies. What does such an examination—a rhetorical understanding of sound in health, healing, and hospital contexts—offer? What does sound mean to health and healing and to whom? When and how do sounds rhetorically transform into power and discipline?

Using Rhetoric to Defy a Sensory Hegemony's Ocular Centrism

Claudius Conrad argued "Music has had an illustrious position in the course of human history: not only as an art, but also as a medium for healing."[32] In ancient Greek medicine, Hippocrates used music to treat mental and physical ailments.[33] Plato and Aristotle agreed that music influenced well-being and healing.[34] However, according to Conrad, Plato thought music could support mental health, and Aristotle held that it could destroy it.[35] When considering that music is made of sound and sound of vibrations, it turns out that these ancient Greek rhetoricians were likely both correct: sound can strengthen health or diminish it—the latter exemplified in Brauer's study of music as torture. In the volume *Sound and the Ancient Senses*, Colin Webster examines "The Soundscape of Ancient Greek Healing."[36] He notes that Hippocratic medical practices thought of "the body as an echoing chamber of noises to be heard, discerned and understood."[37] In misalignment with popularized contemporary Cartesian mind-body binaries that hold science-based, allopathic Western biomedicine's disease-first approaches with drugs and surgeries as treatments as the preeminent health system, Webster claims that we should not accept that there were simply those who used sound—the magico-religious—to treat patients in ancient Greece and those who did not, such as Hippocrates and his students.[38] He asserted that, "From our earliest evidence, music was a part of medicine"[39] (p. 110), which also indicates sound and vibration were as well.

In *Non-Discursive Rhetoric*, Joddy Murray theorizes that rhetoric "must be able to escape the confines of single medium" and "talk[ed] about … as it is experienced …."[40]—an example is @nurse_sushi's description of alarm fatigue. Thomas J. Rickert suggested that "[Rhetoric] must diffuse outward to include material environment, things (including the technological), our own embodiment, and a complex understanding of ecological relationality as participating in rhetorical practices and their theorization."[41] In both instances, Murray and Rickert suggest considering rhetoric outside its common contexts, mediums, and material environments. Jenny Edbauer argues that "An ecological, or *affective*, rhetorical model is one that reads rhetoric both as a process of distributed emergence and as an ongoing circulation process."[42] Edbauer uses the term concatenation—or how things are connected—to describe local ecologies.[43]

What Murray, Rickert, and Edbauer logically assume is the dynamic, affectual, and effectual power of rhetoric that extends beyond once limiting, discursive, bounded, and disconnected notions of it. Underscoring their positions about the power of rhetoric as an analytical approach is the inherent value of acknowledging such connective power. It is an ontological orientation widely—albeit perhaps tacitly—acknowledged and mostly accepted by rhetorical study scholars ("despite a lack of consensus"[44]) evident through the kinds of rhetorical studies scholars undertake. As an example, rhetoric is often explored at the intersection of other concepts, fields, and theories, some material, some not, such as rhetoric and mathematics,[45] rhetoric and disability,[46,47,48] and rhetoric and critical contemporary thought,[49] as well as entire books series (e.g., intersectional rhetoric edited by Karma R. Chávez and transdisciplinary rhetoric edited by Leah Ceccarelli and Michael Bernard-Donals). As Ehren Helmut Pflugfelder points out, claims about rhetoric's expansiveness are not novel,[50] although they might be more newly articulated, especially within RHM.[51]

Recent scholarship from Debra Hawhee,[52] Steph Ceraso,[53] and Emily Winderman, Robert Mejia, and Brendan Rogers[54] (among others) related to sensory rhetorics place our senses near the fore of rhetorical scholarship. Attending to sound in rhetorical field studies uses the "analytical point of departure or arrival"[55] from sound studies, yet theoretically it is complicated, especially when considering available senses. It deprioritizes what S. Scott Graham identified in his study of fibromyalgia as ocular centrism[56] or visualism, which ranks the visual over all other senses. As another example, Winderman, Mejia, and Rogers focused on smell "As an olfactory pedagogy, [that] miasmatism trained the senses to recognize environmentally produced bad smells as threats to individual and collective health"[57]; in turn, their work also contributes to decentering ocular centrism or deprioritizing the visual in (public) health and healing contexts when examined with rhetoric. As a similar function, I suggest prioritizing situated sonicity in fieldwork, even if only temporarily or incompletely, offers an opportunity to counter and perhaps balance what Donna Harraway calls the "much maligned sensory system"[58] vision, or ocular centrism. Harraway in "Situated Knowledges" claims "science—the real game in town—is rhetoric"[59] and that "feminist objectivity is about limited location and situated knowledge."[60] Harraway notes that feminist objectivity "allows us to become answerable for what we learn how to see,"[61] and as I later argue an awareness for what we hear.

However, to be certain, whether prioritizing visual or sound, there are limitations depending on a person's available senses. Winderman, Mejia, and Rogers in "All Smell is Disease: Miasma, Sensory Rhetoric, and the Sanitary-Bacteriologic of Visceral Public Health" make an excellent study of disease as a sight-smell interplay capturing public attention.[62] Although Hawhee seems to caution against parceling the sensorium into discrete senses, such as Winderman, Mejia, and Rogers and myself do, noting "For starters, the idea of the sensorium refuses to separate the senses, to cordon them off into a 'subfield' (e.g., visual studies or sound studies),"[63] it is perhaps ableist and likely inaccurate. Calling upon Alaimo's materialist-feminist concept of trans-corporeality—"the time-space where human corporeality, in all its material fleshiness, is inseparable from 'nature' or 'environment'"[64]—offers an implied plural "body"; Hawhee noted sensorium as "rarely ... plural, it just seems to expand from individual to collective, like breath."[65] Yet, aren't bodies required for sensoria? Do all bodies have all senses? Perhaps a trans-corporeal ethic emerges from sensoria—sensoriums with putative, hegemonic understandings yet "leaky" borders.[66]

Sensoria are vulnerable with unavailable parts to the whole of humanity. In pedagogical contexts, Christina V. Cedillo calls for "critical embodiment" or "approaches that recognize and foreground bodily diversity."[67] Temporarily isolating our sensoria—or viewing all available senses as a complete sensorium—resists sensory hegemony and accounts for real leaky, "living bodies"[68] "unsevered"[69] from rhetoric, sound, health, and healing or better yet wholly and rhetorically considered with rhetoric, sound, health, and healing. Winderman, Mejia, and Rogers showcase an excellent rhetorical investigation of isolating two senses to show how they work together, especially when intersectionally examining historical events through race, class, and gender. In the process, smell is intuited through the visual, yet the visual is not a product of ocular centrism or vision. Instead, the visual amplifies the miasmatic disease etiologies they analyze—typhoid and Zika virus; they also note that "circulating visual rhetoric," such as the images they analyze that represent these two diseases, "implicating smell is central to the sensory transformation of disease systems"[70] because "the visual freezes an olfactory scene."[71] Its absence—the loss of smell or olfaction—captures a common symptom[72] from infection by the SARS-CoV-2 virus or COVID-19 disease. During the pandemic, many infected individuals lost their sense of smell, which also resulted in the loss of normal function of touch and taste or even *chemesthesis*—chemically initiated sensations in mouths.[73] Although clinical reasoning offers scientific explanations for the interplay of our senses (and appear to support Hawhee's caveat to resist separating them), rhetorical examinations, such as Winderman, Mejia, and Rogers, present opportunities to use one sense to prioritize and complement another, especially regarding available senses in various sensoria. In a similar way, as I demonstrate in Chapters 2 and 3, the textual (or visual) preserves the medico-sonic and its use of rhetoric—its "rhetorical circulation"[74] across millennia, cultures, and various health and healing systems.

At some point in history, any mainstay technology, such as a compass, astrolabe, or stethoscope—whether helped by rhetoric or not—requires material and symbolic success.[75] Charles Bazerman acknowledged,

> For any technology to succeed (that is, to establish an enduring place within the world of human activities), it must not only succeed materially (that is, produce specified and reliably repeatable transformations of material and energy); it must also succeed symbolically (that is, adopt significant and stable meanings within germane discourse systems in which the technology is identified, given value, and made the object of human attention and action).[76]

In his rhetorical examination of Edison's inventions and electric light, Bazerman rhetorically situates Edison's invention work among historical and textual evidence to theorize technological success. As I similarly theorize, Laënnec's invention of the stethoscope was successful materially and symbolically—rhetoric situates and powers the stethoscope and medico-sonic knowledge.

Rhetoric is situated, yet rhetoric is expansive, or—better yet—allows expansion. The expansiveness of rhetoric draws from its magnetic, connective power. Edbauer's theorization of rhetorical ecologies demonstrates such power as it "recontextualizes rhetorics in their temporal, historical, and lived fluxes."[77] However, non-discursive, material approaches to rhetoric deprioritize spoken words and texts, such as works by Murray and Rickert. Rhetoric's mutability is powerful in this way; the way it can simultaneously account for the spoken and the unsaid, the seen and unseen, the heard and unheard, the sound and the unsound—the material. It is rhetoric's mutability that makes it expansive, gathering what surrounds it with only the rhetor's, seer's, or listener's discernment. What is caught in rhetoric's net or accounted for in its networks and ecologies can be just as important as what is not. Lisa Melonçon and J. Blake Scott described RHM research expansiveness as "wide-ranging in its topics and their stakeholders,"[78] which makes sense—who isn't touched and what audience isn't engaged by medicine and health and its materiality, especially in times of pandemic? They draw from E. Johanna Hartelius' argument to promote expansiveness as sustainability through sustainable scholarship or "research that offers sound and significant implications for the discipline from which the scholar originally drew his or her theory and method."[79] To reorder several of Hartelius's words, sound offers significant implications; it also offers new understandings of the role of sound in health in healing, theorizations for its exclusion of more ancient health and healing traditions millennia before ancient Rome and Greece, as well as the field research practice concept I offer called sound in all research (SiAR)—an orientation for sonically considering and negotiating embodied research practices and "a unique rhetorical awareness attuned to the material conditions that rhetorical theory may have overlooked"[80] and—from my materialist-feminist perspective—possibly undervalues.

I do not solely examine health and healing from the intersection of rhetoric. In their introduction to the collection *Material Feminisms*, Alaimo and Susan J. Hekman acknowledge from the outset that,

> The purpose ... is to bring the material, specifically the materiality of the human body and the natural world, into the forefront of feminist theory and practice. [...] Materiality, particularly that of bodies and natures, has long been an extraordinarily volatile site for feminist theory ....[81]

My present work aims toward bringing the human body and the natural world to the fore. As an example of my effort, I borrow a term from geography. I examine the *confluence* of rhetoric and sound with bodies, health, and healing across time (Chapters 2–3) and at a specific time (Chapter 4). A confluence or conflux is the merging of two flowing channels of water into one. At the point where they meet, often seeing individuals (such as in Figure 1.1) note two distinctive bodies of water coming together and hearing beings notice the resultant rushing sound from the movement of the joining bodies of water.

Plugfelder calls upon Marback, pointing out that we must "give objects their due"[82] to "understand how things pressure, change, and influence other

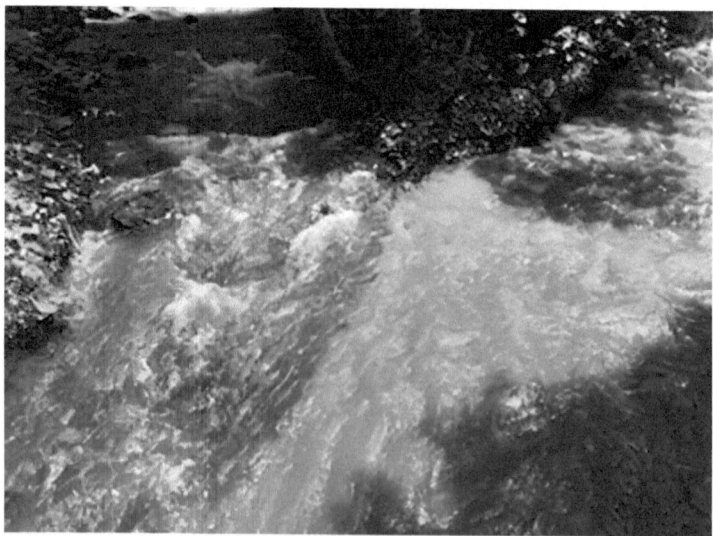

Figure 1.1 Image of two rivers merging near Gstaad in Lauenen, Switzerland (photo by author, 2021).

things and how those relations have lasting impact."[83] Although sound has been underexamined by rhetorical scholars in health, healing, and hospital contexts, it has been addressed in what has been dubbed the sonic turn in rhetorically oriented writing scholarship. Gunn, Goodale, Hall, and Eberly noted in their 2013 review article that sonic studies was "thriving."[84] In her 2016 review of *Rhetoric and Rhythm in Byzantium* by Vesella Valiavitchar-ska, rhetorician and sensory- and body-oriented scholar Hawhee describes that "Scholarship in rhetoric, communication, and communications have very recently seen an uptick in interest in how sound shapes thought, interaction, messages, and sociality."[85] Hawhee goes on to name Goodale, Mathew Jordan, Gunn, Richard Graff, and Jonathan Sterne as leaders of the sonic turn. Amanda Nell Edgar gives sound its due, resisting the "tyranny of the visual," in her material examination of abortion practices that require two corporeal sources of sound: human voice and fetal heartbeat.[86] Her analysis shows the impact of sound by blending rhetoric and sound, theorizing sound's material force, and showing how amplified sound through a healthcare technology is activated to influence action.

Sound, Listening, and Cognition

Heeding Rickert, sonic rhetorician Ceraso makes a case for "multimodal listening."[87-88] Multimodal listening assumes that "sound is not experienced exclusively by a single sense; other parts of the body can be engaged during a sonic encounter."[89] In other words, listening is "full bodied"[90] and a "multisensorial act"[91]—sound works with listeners by engaging aural, visual, and tactile sensibilities—"the synesthetic convergence of sight, sound, and touch,"[92] during (and after) sonic experiences. Ceraso's treatment of listening and listening pedagogy as a multisensorial encounter by the entire body reminds us that sound is experienced through what Hawhee calls an embodied, responsive "mind-body complex"[93]—a concatenation, a conflux of our lived material realities. Influenced by Marshall McLuhan[94] and others, rhetoric's sensorium presumes the interconnectedness of our senses and their sensory ecologies; sonic-visual scholarship from Edgar on reproductive rights, as well as work from Winderman, Mejia, and Rogers on visual-smell and public health demonstrate the value of such sensory examinations in RHM.

For hearing people, sound—not noise (the intention is an important distinction)—is meaningless without the interplay of listening and auditory cognition. Theorizations of listening models[ii] derive from an array of fields,

---

ii Within their context of music and gesture-sound mapping and their contribution of perception-action loop, Baptiste Caramiaux, Jules Françoise, Norbert Schnell, and Frédéric Bevilacqua provide an overview of listening modes spanning nearly 60 years in their article, "Mapping through Listening." They include a taxonomy of listening modes: causal, acoustic, and semantic listening.

such as psychoacoustics, neurosciences, auditory scene analysis, and musicology.[95] Conceptually, I draw from Pierre Schaeffer,[96] R. Murray Schaefer,[97] and Michel Chion,[98] (and primarily Schaefer and Chion) to theorize a sound-listening cognitive interaction in health, healing, and hospital contexts. To start, Schaeffer is widely recognized as providing the first theoretical taxonomy of listening and its functions: (1) listening (*écouter*) or the "indexical value of the sound"; (2) perceiving (*ouïr*) or "receiving the sound, auditorily"; (3) hearing (*entendre*) or attending "to the inherent characteristics of the sound"; and (4) comprehending (*comprendre*) or "bringing in semantics into sounds, treating them as signs."[99] According to Schaeffer, these four listening functions compete yet can occur simultaneously. Building from Schaeffer's taxonomy, Chion classified listening into three categories or modes: causal, reduced, and semantic. *Causal listening* is concerned with determining sources of sounds, while *reduced listening* characterizes sounds, and *semantic listening* interprets sound's messages. His categorizations of hearing are foundational for sound studies and integral for understanding the kind of initial cognitive work listeners perform when they listen. He further described that when a listener is asked about a sound, "their answers are striking for the heterogeneity of levels of hearing to which they refer."[100] From here, I focus on Chion, and I suggest this heterogeneity emanates from listener expertise, cognitive capabilities, and available senses.

Chion describes two levels of causal listening: the first determines a precise cause and the unique source of a sound; the second determines if the sound originates from a human, machine, or animal.[101] For example, take @nurse_ sushi. For healthcare clinicians, it is likely that the precise cause of the alarming monitors tells them that a patient's vital signs have fallen outside a predetermined range. However, for someone without clinical expertise and knowledge, the text that accompanies @nurse_sushi's video's audio is integral to perform that kind of causal listening. Without it, determining that the sound comes from human-machine interaction in general is probably a listener's best guess. Still, these levels of listening are modern descriptions for current understandings—ones with rhetorical roots. Schaefer identifies lo-fi soundscapes—defined as "acoustic [or sonic] environment[s]"[102] perhaps "refer[ring] to actual environments"[103]—that originated in the industrial revolution and resulted in "an overpopulation of sounds" and "… so much acoustical information that little of it can emerge with clarity."[104] For instance, consider the leprosy example. In modern urban soundscapes on a busy street with pedestrian and automobile traffic, would someone approaching either ringing a bell or hitting sticks together be effective or even heard (or seen) if a listener is not in proximity? Chion also reminds that "sound often has not just one source but at least two, three, even more," which can complicate causal listening along with *synchresis*—the confluence or merging of visual and audio.[105]

Reduced listening and semantic listening demand certain cognitive capabilities from the listener. Using Morse code—not entirely unlike the interpretations required of healthcare clinicians listening to healthcare technologies—as an example, Chion describes semantic listening as requiring interpretation based on the integration of spoken language and that code. Chion points out that Schaeffer's reduced listening is the "mode that focuses on the traits of the sound itself, independent of its cause and of its meaning,"[106] which is different from Schaeffer's *ouïr*. Although Chion refers to semantic listening in linguistic contexts for language differences (i.e., phonemes or units of sound), he also notes that listeners can use causal and semantic listening at the same time. By identifying causal or sources of sound in health, healing, and hospital contexts, it is part of my work here to show how rhetoric strategically resides between reduced or characterized and semantic or interpretive listening, as does expertise or what Schafer called "sonological competence"[107]—the unification of "impression with cognition [making] it possible to formulate and express sonic perceptions"—and Chion described as specialist listening. Much of this book inhabits the theoretical space among causal, reduced, and semantic listening and relies on rhetorical devices, such as onomatopoeia, simile, and metaphor, as part of a cognitive process to understand the body's sounds and share those understandings in health, healing, and hospital contexts.

Sonic understandings of bodies have been indexed in medico-sonic lexicons from snippets of translations from ancient Egyptian hieratic script to Laënnec in his foundational *De l'auscultation médiate ou Traité du diagnostic des maladies des poumons et du coeur, fondé principalement sur ce nouveau moyen d'exploration* (or *de l'auscultation médiate* or *of mediated auscultation*). Laënnec's contributions are with us today, as auditory anthropologist Tom Rice[108] and scholars Anna Harris and Melissa Van Drie[109] learned in their sensory-oriented studies about how physicians learn how to auscultate—or use the body's sounds to understand their conditions. Anne Frances Wysocki's "sensuous training"[110] concept posits that "our sensuous perceptions of the world do not just happen 'naturally' but come to their shape in our varying, complex, and socially embedded environments."[111] Rice and Harris and Van Drie describe how physicians receive sensuous training in medical education. Even when intentionally training medical professionals, as Harris and Van Drie argue, there are difficulties because "… educating the senses lies in finding ways to describe and tell about practice and sensory experience,"[112] which is why I argue for rhetoric's substantial role in health, healing, and hospital contexts when interpreting the body's vital functions, as well as foundational for how sound is used diagnostically, prognostically, and therapeutically.

Central to descriptions of sensory experiences are rhetorical mechanisms that draw from common experiences and knowledges to describe what one hears if able. For example, Medzcool is a multimedia resource for students and healthcare professionals; it posted a video on the sounds of coronavirus-infected lungs on YouTube on March 18, 2020.[113] With over 2.1 million views since, the video includes text that describes the context surrounding

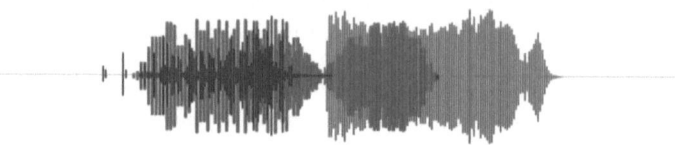

In cases of mild pneumonia, you may auscultate

Fine Crackles (Rales) and Bonchial breath sounds

Fine Crackles
High pitch
Popping sound

Sounds like: firewood burning in a fireplace

Bronchial Sounds
Low pitch
Tubular
Hollow

Figure 1.2 YouTube video from Medzcool stating, "In cases of mild pneumonia, you may auscultate Fine Crackles (Rales) and B[r]onchial breath sounds" (left) and a wave form of the breath sounds above a description of Fine Crackles as "High pitch, Popping sound" and "sounds like firewood burning in a fireplace" and Bronchial sounds as "Low pitch, Tubular; Hollow" (right).

SARS-COV-2 in early 2020, then proceeds to highlight lung or breath sounds associated with COVID-19. It notes that "Early on, breath sounds may sound clear and fast." They describe a "prolonged expiratory phase [that] can be high or low pitched" and as "expiratory wheezing [that is a] continuous [and] musical sound." As shown in Figure 1.2, about 1 minute into the video, the video text states that "In cases of mild pneumonia, you may auscultate [or hear] fine crackles (rales) and bonchial [sic] breath sounds." On the same screen, below a *wave form*—a sound, visualized—of the breath sounds one would hear upon auscultating lungs with a stethoscope or listening to the lungs of a person infected with COVID-19, an image of lungs is on the right screen. Below the waveform, it reads: "fine crackles [:] high pitch popping sound [that] sounds like: firewood burning in a fireplace" and "bronchial sounds [:] low pitch, tubular, hollow."

As the video plays, more text, such as "in extreme cases, COVID-19 can lead to Acute Respiratory Distress syndrome" and "in these cases, breath sounds can appear to sound as distant breath sounds accompanied by coarse rales and diffuse rhonchi" is text paired with the audio of the breath sounds. Coarse crackles are described as having a "low pitch; popping; bubbling" and rhonchi as "continuous; low pitch; rumbling; and gurgling." The Medzcool video uses synchresis and juxtaposes visual text with sound, such as "fine crackles [:] high pitch popping sound [that] sounds like: firewood burning in a fireplace." Medzcool draws from an assumed communal listening experience ("sounds like: firewood burning in a fireplace") and a rhetorical device ("like" signals a simile as the form of comparison) to support shared, reduced listening to make meaning. Causal listening is concerned with determining the source of a sound, which is clearly the lungs amplified via a health technology or stethoscope, while reduced listening characterizes the lung sounds, and semantic listening interprets the sound's messages. Through reduced listening, the sound is characterized and allows an opportunity for semantic listening that interprets the sound's message with rhetorical assistance from a simile ("sounds like: firewood burning in a fireplace"). Without rhetorical devices to assist reduced listening, semantic or expert listening is not likely and medicosonic interplay not possible.

Edbauer's foundational work theorizing rhetorical ecologies also provides an orientation here for understanding the interplay and segmentation of sensory and rhetorical elements within health, healing, and hospital contexts. As Amy Reed points out in her bibliography examining RHM publications between 2000 and 2014, much scholarship in RHM has examined ecological interactions of rhetoric and health.[114] More recently, these interplays of rhetoric and health, medicine, technology have involved the senses. For example, Lillian Campbell and Elizabeth L. Angeli examined and theorized the role of sensory knowledge, situational awareness, and sensory cues or intuition as types of intelligence in clinical nursing and emergency management service simulations for students.[115] By noting how tacit sensory knowledge functions in these contexts, Campbell and Angeli pull in what was seemingly abstract, determine its components, and create a taxonomy for others to understand it. Theirs is an exceptional example of how studies oriented to our senses can function in concatenate health, healing, and hospital contexts when rhetorically oriented.

Katie Lynn Walkup and Peter Cannon orient readers to rhetorical health ecologies to suggest ecological care models for substance abuse treatment to augment mental health literacy and support treatment outcomes.[116] They suggest that a "distributed care framework, power and authority are circulated through patients, providers, technologies, and systems."[117] They also noted that "social and material worlds interact" and "to study one without the other produces an incomplete picture."[118] Their focus on the power of rhetorical health ecologies to "redistribute power and authority"[119] draws upon Edbauer's concept of *rhetorical circulation* to define rhetorical health ecologies as "health ecologies [that] distribute agency through networks of patients and providers."[120] Among other strings of research, they call for future studies to examine how health ecologies affect patient health outcomes, or to put it more simply, how contexts can help or hinder health. I use Edbauer's rhetorical ecologies as an orientation for understanding the interplay and segmentation of sonic and rhetorical elements within health, healing, and hospital contexts—the network or system. Understanding health and healing sites as rhetorically complex, derivative soundscapes, logically recasts them as expansive, yet conceptually bounded spaces within rhetorical ecologies—a kind of what Rice noted in his anthropological and pedagogical study about how physicians learn to listen as a "sensory cross referencing" experience[121] that relies on our experiences, rhetorical and/or actual/otherwise, from without to make sense of within.

Although many scholars have taken up Edbauer's conceptualization of rhetorical ecologies, Robin E. Jensen finds specific value for RHM, noting

> It is this latter focus on rhetorical ecologies of health that I champion ..., not as the only valuable way in which to contribute to conversations within the rhetoric of health but, rather, as a path relatively untrodden and underdeveloped yet teaming with the potential to help decipher the moving target that is 'health' and its related constructs.[122]

Jensen continues, stating: "By attending to health rhetoric's encounters with diverse discursive, sociocultural, and material variables such as affect, this path trades depictions of static rhetorical situations and elements for accounts of rhetorical movement and transformation."[123] The rhetorical situation Jensen proposes is helpful for understanding fluxing knowledge about health and healing—the methodological variety (or mutability[124]) rhetoricians of health and medicine such as myself can draw upon to demonstrate rhetoric's discursive and non-discursive functions and confluences. Edgar offers one such example of rhetorical movement or the confluence of rhetoric, material variables, sound, the body, and healthcare technology—a rhetorical ecology. Edgar notes that although some scholars have focused on visual aspects of sonograms (for example, Carole A. Stabile, Rosalind P. Petchesky, and Julie Roberts), the sonogram was developed from SONAR—a sonic naval technology.[125] Sonography's deployment in abortion and fetal personhood contexts uses the visual and the sonic to produce an "image based on the return of ... sound waves through the [fetal] body, providing a technologically advanced means of listening to interior organs, a technique known as auscultation" and

> while ... Doppler technology ... allows doctors to auscultate fetal heartbeats [it] is not inherently related to the sonogram, they are very often discussed in tandem and linked together in discussion of prenatal examinations and ... mandatory examinations preceding abortions in many states.[126]

Edgar offers an analysis of the "Heartbeat Bill" in Ohio as an example of the rhetorical power of sound in abortion contexts to act as a powerful influence—a "corporeal sound, including the spoken voice and the auscultated heartbeat *as voice* [that] can be understood as material rhetoric, and that material rhetoric, by extension, should be understood as both a force and a networked fluid," "seep[ing] beyond [body] boundaries."[127] Fetal auscultation—the fetal heartbeat—overpowers pregnant voices by amplifying a sonogram's sound, a healthcare technology that relies on sound's material role in our health and healing and an example of the rhetorical power sound wields in health, healing, and hospital contexts. As Edgar effectively demonstrates, amplified bodily sounds are powerful actors with potential to shape actions and experiences.

Pan-Historiography of Sound in Health and Healing

Although I did not set out to write a pan-historiography about sound in health and healing, the expansiveness of rhetoric deposited my curiosity in intellectual and historical places well beyond the boundaries of the NICU from Chapter 4. Two linguistic terms help illuminate the rhetorical-medico-sonic interplay I use to describe my approach: *diachronic*—throughout time—and *synchronic*—specific time. Hawhee and Christa J. Olson also use these terms to describe pan-historiography,[128] which is the rhetorical methodology I use in two chapters. Pan-historiography is the rhetorical method of "writing histories whose temporal scope extends well beyond the span of individual generations"[129] by investigating phenomenon "spread across a vast expanse of time." In Chapters 2 and 3, I use a diachronic approach by looking at the interplay of sound and rhetoric in health and healing contexts "across geographic space, tracking important activities, terms, movements, or practices as they travel ...."[130] Rhetoric's onomatopoeia enabled ancient Egyptians to describe and inscribe the once ineffable sound of a heart's beat as *debdeb*.[131] Then millennia later, Laënnec listened to the body's sounds through a stethoscope and used rhetorical devices to compare a now sonically amplified body with common sounds, such as vesicular respiration sounding like "pair of bellows"—a device used to push out a strong current or blast of air—in his foundational, rhetoric-based text *de l'auscultation médiate*. In part, the broad span of time I cover seeking written descriptions of the body's sounds in various archives represented as rhetorical devices, such as simile and metaphor, works to offer a rhetorical perspective. It also works to argue that the body, sound, and rhetoric can only be partially, not fully severed and understood together as a conflux. To do so, I show how ancient and contemporary physicians interpreted non-discursive sound and used rhetoric to make meaning from it about the body, while drawing from the "materiality of the human body and the natural world"—the once discarded, new material feminist approach Alaimo and Hekman endorse.[132]

Hawhee and Olson primarily explore the challenges and benefits of pan-historiographic approaches; they also note their turn toward the expansive[133]—a potential possibility rhetoric offers—for "a combination of conceptual, theoretical, and practical reasons."[134] By presenting the conflux of sound, rhetoric, and health and healing diachronically and synchronically, I offer a complementary pan (diachronic) and zoom (synchronic) rhetorical view of the phenomenon. The pan-diachronic, zoom-synchronic approach texturizes the other and simultaneously offers breadth and depth; rhetoric helps immensely to develop the concept of SiAR I describe (Chapter 5), while theorizing sound and its relationship with health and healing and pointing out the lived, bodily realities of such a relationship for practical reasons. Through my rhetorical and sonic theorizations of the body and sound, I demonstrate medico-sonic knowledge as an "evolving corporeal practice[e]"[135] and "sprawling history"[136] reliant on rhetoric, non-discursive sound, and the meaning it provokes. In the process, I make possible the "nearly impossible" feminist task of "[engaging] with medicine or science in innovative, productive, or affirmative ways."[137] Hearing and deaf bodies are helped and hurt by sound; the latter—I believe—is unintentional, yet remains harmful, behaving like sonic shrapnel in some health and healing and especially hospital contexts.

Overview of Chapters

In Western biomedical healthcare today, physicians and other healthcare clinicians use percussion and auscultation, along with inspection and palpation, as the four methods to assess the body during a general physical exam.[138] Listening to and amplifying the body's sounds and the functions of its organs, such as the heart, intestines, and lungs, are common clinical practices in conventional, science-based, allopathic Western health systems. By making meaning with the sonic qualities of our bodies from making our bodies sonic, it eventually led to cataloguing and deploying sonic knowledge about bodies in medical education and training, harnessing sonic means through health technologies. I demonstrate how sound and rhetoric "meet across time and place"[139] or have met based on available information. Although my pan-historiographic, diachronic, rhetorical interpretations are not comprehensive or totalizing (and should be thought as such), the NICU at the center of Chapter 4 offers an application of such sonic, synchronic theorizations in a health and healing context, while Chapter 5 more fully considers sonic implications, conceptually and practically.

To start, Chapter 2 provides a touchstone for percussion and auscultation, including more recent contexts for these mainstay medico-sonic bodily assessment tools. Then, using pan-historiography, I rhetorically explore likely origins of medico-sonic practices—from available translated materials—by arguing for the transformation of knowledge about the body's ineffability displayed through onomatopoeia using rhetorical devices in ancient health and healing systems in Mesopotamia, Egypt, India, Greece, and Italy. There are two primary questions explored in this chapter: Historically, how has sound been used in ancient, traditional, and complementary and alternative medicine (CAM) health systems? And how does ineffable bodily sound in health and healing use rhetoric?

In Chapter 3, I identify instances when stethoscope creator Laënnec uses rhetorical devices in his foundational medical education text *de l'auscultation médiate* or *of mediated auscultation* before exploring rhetoric and sound now in health in healing using diagnostic, prognostic, and therapeutic technologies. There are four questions guiding the chapter: How does Laënnec use rhetoric in *de l'auscultation mediate* to create medico-sonic knowledge about the body? How does his use of rhetoric persist today? What modern health and healing technologies use sound diagnostically, prognostically, and therapeutically? How are unintentional uses of sound from healthcare technologies rhetorical?

Chapters 2 and 3 work together to provide a rhetorical version accounting for sound in health in healing, diachronically. An underlying motivation for these chapters is to show a snap shot of deeper, non-European, non-White roots of science-based, allopathic Western biomedicine from available information about ancient health and healing systems. Yet, any history of sound in health and healing, especially based on existing information that remains from the last millennia, erases some contributions through translation, time, or intention. My feminism means drawing attention to what counts, what is worthy of noting or amplifying, which means amplifying a notable absence or omission possibly hindered by past actions and intentions.

Analogous to the rhetorical, pan-historiographies in Chapters 2 and 3, Chapter 4 offers a NICU case study that uses the concept of rhetorical ventriloquism. However, unlike ancient and modern physicians who used other rhetorical devices to develop a medico-sonic system to understand the body's sounds through onomatopoeia, metaphor, and simile, healthcare technologies in Western biomedical healthcare today perform different work, actually and rhetorically. When these healthcare technologies and their soundwaves are rhetorically considered, they sonically display and demonstrate authority and power through these healthcare technologies while performing acts of rhetorical ventriloquism. There is one question guiding Chapter 4: what influence does unintentional sound demonstrate in a hospital context?

The foundation of Chapter 5 emanates from the idea that researchers in health, healing, and hospital contexts should be accountable for what they hear—and can be—by acting as earwitnesses. I contend earwitnessing is a mark of responsible, ethical researcher behavior that contributes to understanding the rhetoric of the "… passively material."[140] The question driving the final chapter arises from a research concept and practice I call SiAR: how can researchers who engage in fieldwork—or individuals who work with those who do—behave responsibly toward sound (or its absence) and its likely effects in research spaces? I offer examples of attending to sound in research spaces. Elsewhere I argued for "prioritizing the bodily experiences of both researcher and participants."[141] By heeding sound and considering its source and impact in field research contexts, we can further dimensionalize and sensorially enrich our data collection, research analyses, findings, and implications. In the process, we can address *sensory hegemony* by resisting ableist ocular centrism,[142] acknowledging sound in research, and reconfiguring vantage points to incorporate sonic dimensions in research. Just as we are responsible for what we see when we conduct fieldwork, we are also responsible for what we hear—Chapter 5 provides a heuristic and practical examples for acting as responsible researchers when conducting fieldwork.

Notes

1 Joshua Gunn, Greg Goodale, Mirko M. Hall, and Rosa A. Eberly. "Auscultating Again: Rhetoric and Sound Studies," *Rhetoric Society Quarterly* 43, no. 5 (2013): 476.

2 Dominic Pettman. *Sonic Intimacy: Voice, Species, Technics (Or, How to Listen to the World)* (Redwood City, CA: Stanford University Press, 2017), 2.

3 Richard Marback. "Unclenching the Fist: Embodying Rhetoric and Giving Objects their Due," *Rhetoric Society Quarterly* 38, no. 1 (2008): 54.

4 Kessler, Molly Margaret. *Stigma Stories: Rhetoric, Lived Experience, and Chronic Illness* (Columbus, OH: The Ohio State University Press, 2022), ix.

5 Ibid., 51.

6 Ibid., 62.

7 Ibid., 31.

8 Ibid., 51.

9 @nurse_sushi. 2021. "Alarm fatigue is high these days #icu #icurn #criticalcare #rn #nurse #covid #covid19 #vaccinessavelives." TikTok, August 19, 2021. https://www.tiktok.com/@nurse_sushi/video/6998078138420890886

10 Katarzyna Lewandowska, Magdalena Weisbrot, Aleksandra Cieloszyk, Wioletta Mędrzycka-Dąbrowska, Sabina Krupa, and Dorota Ozga, "Impact of Alarm Fatigue on the Work of Nurses in an Intensive Care Environment—A Systematic Review," *International Journal of Environmental Research and Public Health* 17, no. 22 (2020): 8409.

11 Sue Sendelbach and Marjorie Funk, "Alarm Fatigue: A Patient Safety Concern," *AACN Advanced Critical Care* 24, no. 4 (2013): 378–86.

12 Ibid., 378.

13 Bradford D. Winters, Maria M. Cvach, Christopher P. Bonafide, Xiao Hu, Avinash Konkani, Michael F. O'Connor, Jeffrey M. Rothschild et al., "Technological Distractions (Part 2): A Summary of Approaches to Manage Clinical Alarms with Intent to Reduce Alarm Fatigue," *Read Online: Critical Care Medicine| Society of Critical Care Medicine* 46, no. 1 (2018): 130–7.

14 Kierra Jones, "Alarm Fatigue a Top Patient Safety Hazard," *Canadian Medical Association Journal* 186, no. 3 (February 2014): 178.

15 Laura Wallis, "Alarm Fatigue Linked to Patient's Death," *American Journal of Nursing* 110, no. 7 (2010): 16.

16 Stacy Alaimo, "Trans-corporeal Feminisms and the Ethical Space of Nature," *Material Feminisms* 25, no. 2 (2008): 238.

17 Schafer, R. Murray, *The Soundscape: Our Sonic Environment and the Tuning of the World* (Simon and Schuster, 1977/1993), 11.

18 Erwin H. Ackerknecht. *A Short History of Medicine* (Baltimore, MD: JHU Press, 2016), 106.

19 Donald G. McNeil Jr, "Fast New Test Could Find Leprosy Before Damage Is Lasting," *The New York Times,* February 19, 2013. https://www.nytimes.com/2013/02/20/health/fast-new-test-could-help-nip-leprosy-in-the-bud.html

20 Luke Demaitre. "The Clapper as 'vox miselli': New Perspectives on Iconography," in *Leprosy and identity in the Middle Ages*, eds. Elma Brenner and François-Olivier Touati (Manchester, UK: Manchester University Press, 2021), 208–66.

21 Kristin M. Bivens, Lora Arduser, Candice A. Welhausen, and Michael J. Faris. "A Multisensory Literacy Approach to Biomedical Healthcare Technologies: Aural, Tactile, and Visual Layered Health Literacies," *Kairos*, 22 no. 2 (2018). https://kairos.technorhetoric.net/22.2/topoi/bivens-et-al/index.html

22 Jonathan Sterne, *The Audible Past* (Durham, NC: Duke University Press, 2003), 492, https://doi.org/10.1515/9780822384250-toc.

23 François Cooren. "The Selection of Agency as a Rhetorical Device: Opening up the Scene of Dialogue through Ventriloquism." *Dialogue and Rhetoric* (2008): 23–37.
24 Ibid., 23–24.
25 Stacy Alaimo, "Trans-corporeal Feminisms and the Ethical Space of Nature," 242.
26 Cindy Boren. "Four Skiers Killed in Utah, Bringing U.S. Avalanche Death Toll to 21 this Season," *The Washington Post*, February 7, 2021. https://www.washingtonpost.com/sports/2021/02/07/utah-avalanche-kills-skiers/
27 Kenneth C. Balcomb III. *Sonic Sea* (Natural Resources Defense Council, 2016), 60 minutes. https://www.sonicsea.org/
28 Juliane Brauer. "How Can Music Be Torturous? Music in Nazi Concentration and Extermination Camps," *Music & Politics* 10, no. 1 (2016): 1.
29 Ibid., 2.
30 Ibid., 6.
31 R. Murray Schafer. *The Soundscape: Our Sonic Environment and the Tuning of the World* (New York: Simon and Schuster, 1993), 272.
32 Claudius Conrad. "Music for Healing: From Magic to Medicine," *The Lancet* 376, no. 9757 (2010): 1980.
33 Christof F. Kleisiaris, Christos F., Chrisanthos Sfakianakis, and Ioanna V. Papathanasiou. "Health Care Practices in Ancient Greece: The Hippocratic Ideal," *Journal of Medical Ethics and History of Medicine* 7 (2014), 6–10.
34 Ibid.
35 Ibid.
36 Colin Webster, "The Soundscape of Ancient Greek Healing," in *Sound and the Ancient Senses*, eds. Shane Butler and Sarah Nooter (London, UK: Routledge, 2018), 109–29.
37 Ibid., 109.
38 Ibid., 112.
39 Ibid., 110.
40 Joddy Murray, *Non-Discursive Rhetoric: Image and Affect in Multimodal Composition* (Albany, NY: SUNY Press, 2009), 2.
41 Thomas Rickert, *Ambient Rhetoric: The Attunements of Rhetorical Being* (Pittsburgh, PA: University of Pittsburgh Press, 2013), 3.
42 Jenny Edbauer, "Unframing Models of Public Distribution: From Rhetorical Situation to Rhetorical Ecologies," *Rhetoric Society Quarterly* 35, no. 4 (2005): 13; emphasis original.
43 Ibid., 22.
44 Gunn, Greg, Hall, and Eberly, Auscultating again, 476.
45 James Wynn and G. Mitchell Reyes, eds. *Arguing with Numbers: The Intersections of Rhetoric and Mathematics*. Vol. 16. (University Park, PA: Penn State Press, 2021).
46 Christina V. Cedillo, "What Does It Mean to Move?: Race, Disability, and Critical Embodiment Pedagogy." *Composition Forum* 39 (2018). https://compositionforum.com/issue/39/to-move.php
47 Kessler. *Stigma Stories*.
48 Lisa Melonçon. *Rhetorical Accessability: At the Intersection of Technical Communication and Disability Studies* (New York: Routledge, 2014).
49 Omar Swartz. *The Rise of Rhetoric and Its Intersection with Contemporary Critical Thought* (New York: Routledge, 2019).
50 Ehren Helmut Pflugfelder, "Rhetoric's New Materialism: From Micro-rhetoric to Microbrew," *Rhetoric Society Quarterly* 45, no. 5 (2015): 442.
51 J. Blake Scott and Lisa Melonçon. "Expansiveness in/through RHM," *Rhetoric of Health & Medicine* 2, no. 1 (2019): iii–ix.

52 Debra Hawhee, Rhetoric's Sensorium, *Quarterly Journal of Speech*, 101, no. 1 (2015): 2–17.

53 Steph Ceraso, *Sounding Composition: Multimodal Pedagogies for Embodied Listening* (Pittsburgh, PA: University of Pittsburgh Press, 2018).

54 Emily Winderman, Robert Mejia, and Brandon Rogers. "All Smell is Disease": Miasma, Sensory Rhetoric, and the Sanitary-Bacteriologic of Visceral Public Health," *Rhetoric of Health & Medicine* 2, no. 2 (2019): 115–46.

55 Jonathan Sterne, ed., *The Sound Studies Reader* (New York: Routledge, 2012), 2, https://ia800308.us.archive.org/10/items/orejainculta-antropologia-sonora/14. Sterne_the%20sound%20studies%20reader.pdf.

56 S. Scott Graham "Agency and the Rhetoric of Medicine: Biomedical Brain Scans and the Ontology of Fibromyalgia," *Technical Communication Quarterly* 18, no. 4 (2009): 376–404.

57 Winderman, Mejia, Rogers, "All Smell is Disease," 116.

58 Donna Harraway, "Situated Knowledges: The Science Question in Feminism and the Privilege of Partial Perspective," *Feminist Studies* 14, no. 3, 581.

59 Ibid., 577.

60 Ibid., 583.

61 Ibid., 583.

62 Winderman, Mejia, Rogers, "All Smell is Disease," 115–46.

63 Debra Hawhee. "Rhetoric's Sensorium," *Quarterly Journal of Speech* 101, no. 1 (2015): 2–17.

64 Alaimo, "Trans-corporeal Feminisms and the Ethical Space of Nature," 238.

65 Hawhee, "Rhetoric's Sensorium," 5.

66 Alaimo, "Trans-corporeal Feminisms and the Ethical Space of Nature," 262.

67 Cedillo, "What Does It Mean to Move?," n.p.

68 Ibid.

69 Alaimo, "Trans-corporeal Feminisms and the Ethical Space of Nature, 262.

70 Winderman, Mejia, and Rogers, "All Smell is Disease," 121.

71 Ibid., 122.

72 Michael Marshall. "COVID's Toll on Smell and Taste: What Scientists Do and Don't Know," *Nature* 589, no. 7842 (2021): 342–3.

73 Marshall, "COVID's toll on smell and taste," 342.

74 Winderman, Mejia, and Rogers, "All Smell is Disease," 138.

75 Charles Bazerman. *The Languages of Edison's Light* (Cambridge, MA: MIT Press, 1999).

76 Bazerman, *The Languages of Edison's Light*, 335.

77 Edbauer, "Unframing Models of Public Distribution," 9.

78 Scott and Melonçon, "Expansiveness in/through RHM," iii.

79 E. Johanna Hartelius, Review Essay: Sustainable Scholarship and the Rhetoric of Medicine, *Quarterly Journal of Speech*, 95, no. 4 (2009): 466.

80 Pflugfelder, "Rhetoric's New Materialism," 442.

81 Stacy Alaimo and Susan J. Hekman, eds. *Material Feminisms* (Bloomington, IN: Indiana University Press, 2008), 1.

82 Richard Marback. "Unclenching the Fist: Embodying Rhetoric and Giving Objects their Due." *Rhetoric Society Quarterly* 38, no. 1 (2008): 46–65

83 Pflugfelder, "Rhetoric's New Materialism," 442.

84 Gunn, Joshua, Greg Goodale, Mirko M. Hall, and Rosa A. Eberly, "Auscultating Again: Rhetoric and Sound Studies," *Rhetoric Society Quarterly* 43, no. 5 (2013): 476.

85 Debra Hawhee. "Review of Rhetoric and Rhythm in Byzantium: The Sound of Persuasion," *Rhetorica*, 34, no. 4 (2018): 466.

86 Amanda Nell Edgar. "The Rhetoric of Auscultation: Corporeal Sounds, Mediated Bodies, and Abortion Rights," *Quarterly Journal of Speech* 103, no. 4 (2017): 351.
87 Steph Ceraso. "(Re) Educating the Senses: Multimodal Listening, Bodily Learning, and the Composition of Sonic Experiences," *College English* 77, no. 2 (2014): 102–23.
88 Ibid.
89 Ibid., 102.
90 Ibid., 103.
91 Ibid., 102.
92 Ibid., 104.
93 Debra Hawhee. "Rhetoric's Sensorium." *Quarterly Journal of Speech* 101, no. 1 (2015): 10.
94 Marshall McLuhan. *Understanding Media: The Extensions of Man* (Cambridge, MA: MIT Press, 1994).
95 Baptiste Caramiaux, Jules Françoise, Norbert Schnell, and Frédéric Bevilacqua, "Mapping through Listening," *Computer Music Journal* 38, no. 3 (2014): 34–48.
96 Caramiaux, Françoise, Schnell, and Bevilacqua, "Mapping through Listening."
97 R. Murray Schafer, *The Soundscape: Our Sonic Environment and the Tuning of the World* (Rochester, VT: Destiny Books, 1977/1994).
98 Michel Chion. "The Three Listening Modes," in *The Sound Studies Reader*, ed. Jonathan Sterne (London, UK: Routledge, 2012), 48–53.
99 Caramiaux, Françoise, Schnell, and Bevilacqua, "Mapping through Listening,"36.
100 Chion, "The Three Listening Modes," 48.
101 Ibid., 48–49
102 Schafer, *The Soundscape*, 7.
103 Ibid., 274.
104 Ibid., 71.
105 Chion, "The Three Listening Modes," 49.
106 Ibid., 50.
107 Schafer, *The Soundscape*, 274.
108 Tom Rice, "Learning to Listen: Auscultation and the Transmission of Auditory Knowledge," *Journal of the Royal Anthropological Institute* 16 (2010): S41, http://www.jstor.org/stable/40606064.
109 Anna Harris and Melissa Van Drie, "Sharing Sound: Teaching, Learning, and Researching Sonic Skills," *Sound Studies* 1, no. 1 (2015): 98–117.
110 Anne Frances Wysocki, Unfitting Beauties of Transducing Bodies. In Stuart A. Selber, ed, *Rhetorics and Technologies: New Directions in Writing and Communication*, (Columbia, SC: University of South Carolina Press, 2010), 94–112.
111 Ibid., 104.
112 Harris and Van Drie, "Sharing Sound," 98.
113 Medzcool. "Sounds of Coronavirus (COVID-19) – Lung Sounds. YouTube, March 18, 2020, https://www.youtube.com/watch?v=3Kkp6ZM35As
114 Amy R. Reed, "Building on Bibliography: Toward Useful Categorization of Research in Rhetorics of Health and Medicine," *Journal of Technical Writing and Communication* 48, no. 2 (2018): 175–198.
115 Lillian Campbell and Elizabeth L. Angeli. "Embodied Healthcare Intuition: A Taxonomy of Sensory Cues Used by Healthcare Providers," *Rhetoric of Health & Medicine* 2, no. 4 (2019): 353–83.
116 Katie Lynn Walkup and Peter Cannon. "Health Ecologies in Addiction Treatment: Rhetoric of Health and Medicine and Conceptualizing Care," *Technical Communication Quarterly* 27, no. 1 (2018): 108–20.
117 Ibid., 108.

118 Ibid., 111.
119 Ibid., 112.
120 Ibid., 112.
121 Rice, "Learning to Listen," S50.
122 Robin E. Jensen, "An Ecological Turn in Rhetoric of Health Scholarship: Attending to the Historical Flow and Percolation of Ideas, Assumptions, and Arguments," *Communication Quarterly* 63, no. 5 (2015): 523.
123 Ibid., 523.
124 Lisa Melonçon and J. Blake Scott, eds. *Methodologies for the Rhetoric of Health & Medicine* (New York: Taylor & Francis, 2018), 5.
125 Edgar, "The Rhetoric of Auscultation," 1–2.
126 Ibid., 2.
127 Ibid., 2. Emphasis original.
128 Debra Hawhee and Christa J. Olson. "Pan-historiography: The Challenges of Writing History across Time and Space," in *Theorizing Histories of Rhetoric*, ed. Michelle Ballif (Carbondale, IL: Southern Illinois University Press, 2013), 90–105.
129 Ibid., 90.
130 Ibid.
131 Bernard Ziskind and Bruno Halioua, "Les Égyptiens sont-ils les pionniers de l'auscultation?," *La Presse Médicale* 32, no. 32 (2003): 1507.
132 Alaimo and Hekman, *Material Feminisms*.
133 Hawhee and Olson, "Pan-historiography," 95.
134 Ibid.
135 Alaimo and Henkman, *Material Feminisms*, 3.
136 Hawhee and Olson, "Pan-historiography," 91.
137 Alaimo and Henkman, *Material Feminisms*, 4.
138 "Assessing Patients Effectively: Here's How to Do the Basic Four Techniques," *Nursing* 8, no. 2 (November 2006): 6, https://journals.lww.com/nursing/Fulltext/2006/11002/Assessing_patients_effectively__Here_s_how_to_do.5.aspx.
139 Hawhee and Olson, "Pan-historiography," 97.
140 Rickert, *Ambient Rhetoric*, 3.
141 Bivens, Kristin Marie. "Rhetorically Listening for Microwithdrawals of Consent in Research Practice," in *Methodologies for the Rhetoric of Health & Medicine,*, eds. Lisa Melonçon and J. Blake Scott pp. 138–156 (New York: Routledge, 2017), 147.
142 Graham, S. Scott, "Agency and the Rhetoric of Medicine: Biomedical Brain Scans and the Ontology of Fibromyalgia," *Technical Communication Quarterly* 18, no. 4 (2009): 376–404.

2 A Sonic Lineage of Percussion and Auscultation from Ancient Mesopotamian, Egyptian, Indian, Greek, and Roman Medicine

Anthropologist and sonic studies scholar Shannon Mattern characterized the body as a "resonance chamber whose particular sonic qualities can reveal its condition of well-being."[1] In this chapter, I account for the ancient, the enduring, and the once novel methods to understand the body's sonic qualities with rhetoric. Making the body's sounds and its resonance chamber properties meaningful is enabled by the non-discursive, such as the *beat beat beat* or the ancient Egyptian "*debdeb*" of our hearts and the sound of air moving through our lungs or intestines. These sounds provide *medico-sonic* information— bodily sounds systematically interpreted through medical knowledge mediated by rhetoric and the medical use of the sounds of our bodies and sound on our bodies. Medico-sonic physiological sounds, sometimes represented via onomatopoeia, were once *ineffable*—or unable to be put into words—until modern physicians used other rhetorical devices to develop medico-sonic systems to understand the body's sounds. It is commonly thought that modern physicians, starting with Austrian Joseph Leopold von Auenbrügger's tapping or percussion method and French René Theophile-Hyacinthe Laënnec's invention of the stethoscope in 1816, ushered the advent of harnessing the body's sounds to make sense of its physiological processes; however, physicians and others who have cared for people's health have used unaided ears and the body's sound to care for others throughout available recorded human history.

Perhaps surprisingly (or not), figures of speech and the rhetorical affordances provided through similes and standard metaphors were the physician's tools that moved the ineffable sounds and noises of the body from onomatopoeia—*debdeb*—to evocative descriptions using similes, such as a lung that sounds "as if it were boiling inside like vinegar"[2]—Hippocrates of Kos's (who lived around 2,500 years ago)[3] description of lung or breath sounds made after placing his unaided ear on a patient's chest[4]—or to Laënnec's "a tinkling, like that of a small bell which has just stopped ringing, or of a gnat buzzing within a porcelain vase."[5] These foundational, yet developing medico-sonic descriptions and eventual categorizations of the body's sounds ultimately evolved into widely shared medico-sonic knowledge with bodily based acoustical nomenclature. Physician-cum-translators, like Laënnec's

DOI: 10.4324/9781032724416-2

teacher Jean-Nicolas Corvisart who translated Auenbrügger's foundational work on percussion from Latin to French or John Forbes who translated Laënnec's groundbreaking work on auscultation from French to English, adventitiously expedited the use of sound in clinical physical examinations. Translations are rhetorical endeavors mediated by biases, assumptions, and even cultural expectations, especially when modern readers rely on translated interpretations of ancient cuneiform and hieratic script, or certain cultural subjectivities revealed through rhetorical devices like simile and metaphor from foregone civilizations many thousands of years ago.

Using Jenny Edbauer's distributed rhetorical ecologies and an understanding that "rhetorical situations involve the amalgamation and mixture of many different events and happenings that are not properly segmented into audience, text, or rhetorician,"[6] translated, fragmented sonic examples scattered across time among ancient health and healing systems demonstrate that although improperly segmented, these sonic examples currently inhabit an established, widely used medico-sonic ecology. Accelerating in the last two centuries, with the use of sound to signal an alarm for the body's respiratory, circulatory, and digestive processes, the metamorphosis was gradual for several millennia prior, including millennia before the common era (BCE), and—as I argue—enabled and augmented by rhetoric. To show a rhetorical, sonic transformation, I rely on Debra Hawhee and Christa J. Olson's methodology pan-historiography[7] to trace the body's sounds and the clinical interpretation of "audible signs of disease within the body"[8] by naked and likely unaided ears from scattered, translated examples of auscultation and percussion in ancient health systems. I argue for the transformation of knowledge about the body's ineffability (i.e., onomatopoeia) by rhetorical devices (i.e., simile and metaphor)—making meaning with the sonic qualities of our bodies from making our bodies sonic—that eventually led to cataloguing and deploying sonic knowledge about bodies in medical education and training, harnessing, and transducing sonic means through health technologies powered by rhetoric.

Acoustic Traces of Bodily Processes: Percussion and Auscultation

In *science-based, allopathic Western biomedicine*—the predominant medical system that treats symptoms and diseases with drugs, interventions, and operations—today, physicians and other healthcare clinicians use percussion and auscultation, along with inspection and palpation, as the four methods to assess the body during general physical exams.[9] Listening to and amplifying the body's sounds and the functions of its organs, such as the heart, intestines, and lungs, are common clinical practices in modern medicine. As auditory anthropologist Tom Rice put it, "sounds that doctors interpret using auscultation could be understood as the acoustic traces of bodily processes."[10] In some way, each of these physical examination assessment methods involves hearing or listening to and interpreting the body's physiological sounds. However, there is evidence from cuneiform and hieratic script and Sanskrit translations from ancient medical systems indicating—over 5,000 years ago—physicians used the body's sounds to assess and diagnose through percussion and auscultation.

Percussion (Latin: *percussio*) includes "tapping your fingers or hands quickly and sharply against parts of the patient's body to locate organ borders, identify organ shape and position, and determine if an organ is solid or filled with fluid or gas," and indirect percussion uses sound to provide clues that might help determine an underlying tissue's form.[11] Auscultation (Latin: *ausculto*) involves listening to breath as it moves through the lungs, the heart as it pumps to circulate blood throughout the body, and abdominal sounds that can indicate intestinal health. Whether we listen or not, the body's sonic qualities disclose much about us.

Percussion

Percussion—as its name implies—involves striking something to produce a noise, and it relies on a particular body part to produce a sound.[12] "Assessing Patients Effectively" describes percussion as "tapping your fingers or hands quickly and sharply against parts of the patient's body to help you locate organ borders, identify organ shape and position, and determine if an organ is solid or filled with fluid or gas."[13] In tandem with inspection, but performed after auscultation, yet before palpation, percussion involves using one's digits, hands, or even a small implement to determine

- the size, consistency, and borders of body organs; and
- the presence or absence of fluid in body areas.[14]

To the trained, sonologically competent ear, the resultant "sound is a sign of the type of tissue within the body part or organ."[15] For example, if a lung sounds hollow, the lung is full of air. Or, while bones, joints, and some organs sound solid, the abdomen "sounds like a hollow organ filled with air, fluid, or solids."[16] There are two types of percussion: *direct*—with one or two fingers—and *indirect*—with the middle or flexor finger. To produce a meaningful sound open to clinical interpretation, the latter is used to "give clues to the makeup of the underlying tissue."[17]

Auscultation

Usually, a stethoscope assists in the clinical physical exam technique known as auscultation, which means "to listen." *Immediate auscultation* means an ear is placed directly to a person's chest (as in Figure 2.1), while *mediate auscultation* uses a stethoscope or auscultates via portable Doppler (with a handheld

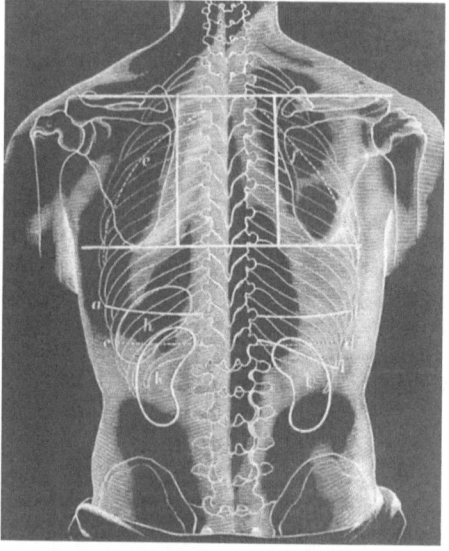

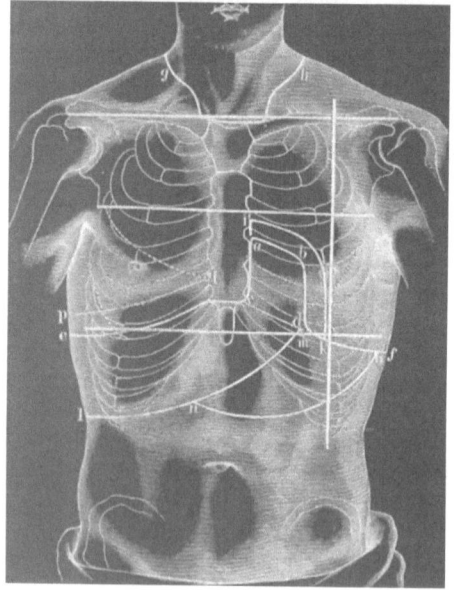

Figure 2.1 Modified images from pages 42–43 of *A Manual of Auscultation and Percussion: Embracing the Physical Diagnosis of Diseases of the Lungs and Heart, and of Thoracic Aneurysm* (Philadelphia: Lea Brothers & Co., 1890)[20] that shows the organ boundaries and areas where physicians and healthcare clinicians auscultate and percuss patients during clinical physical examinations from the back (top) and from the front (bottom).

ultrasound transducer). Listening to the body through auscultation has been described by Rice as listening to "the acoustic traces of bodily processes"[18] that only those with sonological competence or clinical training and expertise can interpret. For example, if a nurse or physician were to use a stethoscope to perform mediate auscultation to assess a person, they would rely on their clinical skills to perform the following tasks:

- Use the diaphragm to pick up high-pitched sounds, such as first (S1) and second (S2) heart sounds. Hold the diaphragm firmly against the patient's skin, using enough pressure to leave a slight ring on the skin afterward.
- Use the [stethoscope's] bell to pick up low-pitched sounds, such as third (S3) and fourth (S4) heart sounds. Hold the bell lightly against the patient's skin, just hard enough to form a seal. Holding the bell too firmly causes the skin to act as a diaphragm, obliterating low-pitched sounds.
- Listen to and try to identify the characteristics of one sound at a time.[19]

For certain, assessing patients via stethoscopic auscultation relies upon experiences derived from listening and interpreting the sounds of the body, as Rice describes in his study of cardiac listening via mediated auscultation in medical school training.[21] Auscultation, though, is an ancient medical practice. As the following sections show, clinically using the body's sounds to understand its physical condition is an ancient, long-held practice spanning multiple continents and several millennia. Rice argues that mediated auscultation through a stethoscope is a "practice which might otherwise be subsumed by, or regarded as merely another technique embedded within, a more encompassing medical habitus"[22]; however, sound and listening to the body are part of its ancient allopathic lineage[23]—one that I use pan-historiography to *redescribe*[i] as rhetorical. To demonstrate sound's mainstay presence and prominence in health and healing, I provide an overview of diagnostic and therapeutic sound from an array of health systems (ancient and conventional medicine, as well as CAM modalities). By demonstrating several of sound's present and historical uses in health and healing, I set the stage to move my argument forward in Chapter 3 that some sounds and their uses in health and healing are intentional, diagnostic, prognostic, or therapeutic, while some sounds in health and healing are unintentional, yet persuasive, and thus rhetorical. As I later articulate, rhetoric powers minimally regulated, unintentional sound as it circulates—with or without intended purpose—and disrupts and disciplines in the process.

---

i I use *redescribe* in the same sense as sound studies scholar Jonathan Sterne: "I say it redescribes rather than describes because good scholarship always goes beyond the common-sense categories used in everyday descriptive language—it tells us what we don't already know" (Jonathan Sterne, ed., *The Sound Studies Reader* [New York: Routledge, 2012], 2, https://ia800308.us.archive.org/10/items/orejainculta-antropologia-sonora/14.Sterne_the%20sound%20studies%20reader.pdf).

To frame the rhetorical move from ineffable rhetoric to establishing sound as disrupting and disciplining, several questions are answered throughout this chapter:

• Historically, how has sound been used in ancient and CAM health systems?
• How is ineffable bodily sound in health and healing powered by rhetoric?

By describing several ancient, notable, and knowable examples of sound in health and healing, I demonstrate the sonic lineage of modern medico-sonic knowledge when mediated by rhetoric. Like Hawhee and Olsen, through pan-historiography, I endeavor to "enliven and physicalize"[24] by "reanimating ... in a way that renders visible, audible, and lively"[25] the sound in ancient health and healing systems. By doing so, I set up the next chapter, which is organized into four sections: diagnostic, prognostic, therapeutic, and unintentional sound in health and healing, which moves us toward the current day.

Interpreting the Body's Sounds: From Auenbrügger's Percussion and Laënnec's Auscultation to Perduring Sound from Ancient Health and Healing Systems

Although reified in allopathic Western health systems and taught throughout biomedical and clinical education and training, percussion and auscultation have deeper medico-sonic roots than from their codified practice in the last few hundred years. Starting with percussion and its modern introduction in *Inventum Novum ex Percussione Thoracis Humani ut Signo Abstrusos Interni Pectoris Morbos Detegendi* (*A New Discovery that Enables the Physician from the Percussion of the Human Thorax to Detect the Diseases Hidden Within the Chest*, 1761), Austrian physician Auenbrügger is thought to be responsible for introducing percussion as a diagnostic technique. However, even in Auenbrügger's time, other physicians thought he had plagiarized percussion from Hippocrates, and *Inventum Novum* received "unfavorable and even hostile reviews."[26] In fact, what is known about ancient Greek or humoral medicine, the writings and translations of which scholars of health and medicine might be familiar, is primarily attributed to Hippocrates (c. 460–c. 370 BCE).[27] According to Rachel Hajar in "The Art of Listening," "Hippocrates advocated for the search of practical instruments to improve medicine in 350 BC. He discussed a procedure for shaking a patient by the shoulders (succussion) and listening for sounds evoked by the chest."[28]

Although drawing upon vibration in similar ways to Hippocrates, Auenbrügger's percussion technique was different. As a method of clinical diagnosis, percussion was not immediately or widely practiced. In Alex Sakula's approximation, Auenbrügger's percussion was a "new method of clinical examination for detection of lung consolidation, pleural effusion, and so on."[29]

H. Kenneth Walker described Corvisart as "France's greatest clinician" who recognized value in Auenbrügger's percussion method as a physician's tool for physical assessment of patients.[30] When Corvisart translated *Inventum Novum* into English from Latin, he included 20 years of his findings of using percussion clinically.[31] Corvisart later taught percussion to Laënnec during his medical training in France, and percussion became more widely used and accepted.[32] In fact, Laënnec devoted Chapter 2 of *Traité de l'auscultation médiate et des maladies des poumons et du cœur* (*A Treatise on the Diseases of the Chest and on Mediate Auscultation* or *de l'auscultation médiate*) to percussion. At the outset of the chapter, Laënnec wrote,

> The chest of a healthy person when slightly struck, ought to yield over its whole extent, more particularly in its anterior and lateral parts, a clear and distinct sound, owing to the presence of the air, which constantly fills the lungs, and consequently a great portion of the cavity of the thorax.[33]

Within the chapter, Laënnec refers to Auenbrügger and his percussion method multiple times.

Prior to Laënnec's invention of the stethoscope in 1816, immediate auscultation—or listening to the body's organs and their functions—required the listener to put their ear near or directly on the patient's body (see Figure 2.2) while the listener tried to hear heart, intestine, and lung sounds for their expert clinical interpretation. Before the stethoscope, according to Hajar, "Hippocrates also used the method of applying the ear directly to the chest and found it useful in order to detect the accumulation of fluid within the chest."[34] Since the early 19th century, for example, lung sounds might be described as high or low pitched and accompanied by wheezing or crackling. Or percussion of the abdomen might indicate whether the cavity is gas-, fluid-, or solid-filled. Whatever the sound, with training and expert applications of F. Murray Schaefer's sonological competence or Michel Chion's semantic listening, those clinical exam sounds, and subsequent interpretations, suggest diagnoses and indicate therapeutic treatments.

According to Laënnec, feeling the heart through "the application of the hand to the region of the heart was, for a long time, the chief means employed by the ancient physicians to judge of the strength, weakness, or other characters [sic] of the pulse."[36] Immediate or direct auscultation "had been known, but little practised, [sic] from ancient times."[37] There were other issues related to immediate auscultation that likely prompted Laënnec's invention of the stethoscope, such as it "was uncomfortable for the patient and the physician, indelicate and impractical in women, and not hygienic."[38] In the late 18th and early 19th centuries, it is estimated that about one-quarter of the population died from tuberculosis.[39] Since Laënnec studied this pulmonary disease—the same disease from which his mother died (at age 32) and to which his uncle, younger brother, teacher Xavier Bichat (at age 31), and great friend Gaspard Laurent Bayle (at age 42) eventually succumbed[40]—the

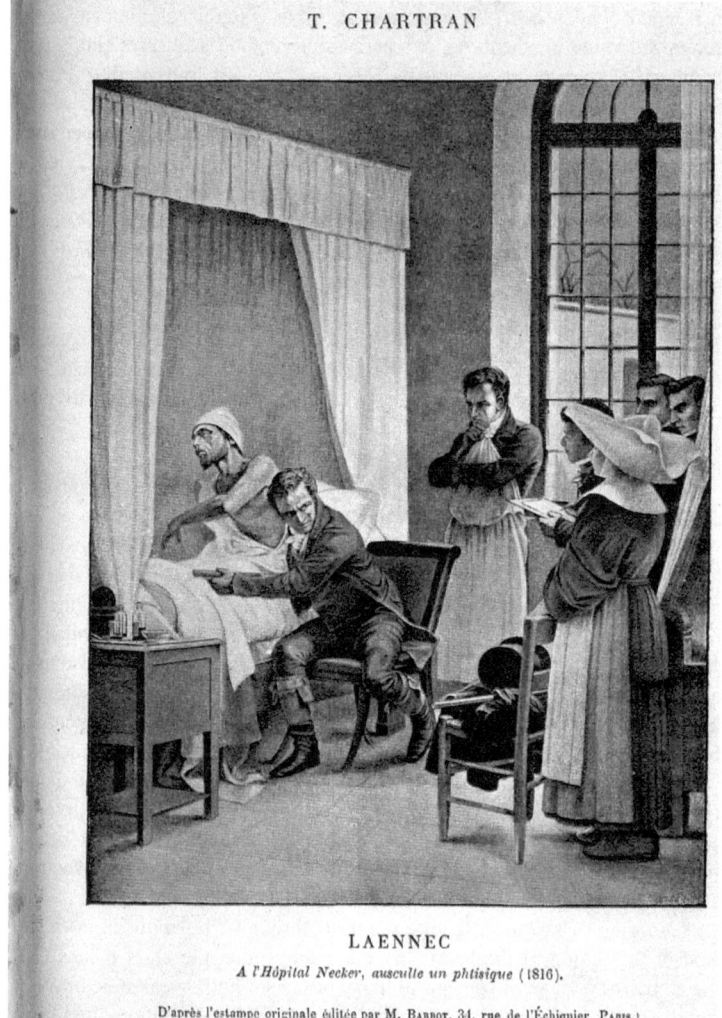

T. CHARTRAN

LAENNEC

A l'Hôpital Necker, ausculte un phtisique (1816).

D'après l'estampe originale éditée par M. Barror, 34, rue de l'Échiquier, Paris.)

Figure 2.2 In the same year he is credited with creating the stethoscope, Laënnec lis-
tens or uses immediate auscultation on a patient at the Necker Hospital in
Paris. *Laënnec à l'hôpital Necker ausculte un phtisique devant ses élèves*
(1816) by Théobald Chartran (1849–1907).[35]

issue of hygiene was likely a reasonable concern. Laënnec himself would die from *phthisis pulmonalis*, or tuberculous, by age 45.[41] In a preface to his translation of Laënnec's treatise, Forbes writes, "It is somewhat curious that he shared the fate of some of his most illustrious predecessors, in falling a victim to a disease, the nature of which he had taken particular pains to illustrate."[42]

Laënnec's nearly 500-page *de l'auscultation médiate* is thought of "as the pioneer treatise from which modern chest medicine has evolved."[43] Along with *de l'auscultation médiate*, Laënnec furnished handcrafted wooden stethoscopes he made to accompany those copies.[44] No doubt this practice of selling stethoscopes with the text that explained how to use them helped users understand the stethoscope's applications. Since Laënnec described the sounds of lungs, both normal and abnormal, as heard via mediate auscultation by stethoscope, it provided immediate opportunities for other physicians to test Laënnec's work. Forbes's translation of Laënnec's catalogue of the body's once ineffable sounds—mediated by the stethoscope and interpreted and tested through medical training—uses rhetorical devices like simile and metaphor to create a medico-sonic directory of the body's sounds. For instance, "like that of the sea" or "produced by the application of a large shell to the ear" to describe a heart murmur.[45] Throughout *de l'auscultation médiate*, Laënnec extended beyond onomatopoeia and used rhetorical devices to redescribe the body's ineffable sounds as sonic and widely knowable.

Although Laënnec's categorizations rely on simile and metaphor to make meaning of the body's sounds, he also classifies the body's sounds, like the simile and metaphor for a heart murmur, into broader categories. For example, Laënnec described various heart or cardiac sounds:

> On the other hand, when the ventricular parietes are thin, the sound produced by their contraction is clear and loud, approaching to that of the auricles; and if there be a marked dilatation of the ventricles, the sound becomes nearly similar, and almost as strong as that of the auricles. In the case of considerable dilatation, the two sounds can be distinguished, the impulse of the heart has been perceived.[46]

And,

> The heart and arteries, under certain circumstances, in place of the sound which naturally attends their dilatation, produce what I have denominated the *bellows-sound*, from the circumstance of its exactly resembling, in the greater number of cases at least, the noise produced by this instrument when used to blow the fire.[47]

For sonic understandings of the body's health and function, Laënnec's *de l'auscultation médiate* is perhaps rhetorically unsurpassed in its novel, cognitively and aurally orienting, medico-sonic work. In his chapter "Sonic Imaginations," Jonathan Sterne noted that "particular ways of knowing sound have been integral to the development of key modern sonic practices"[48]; I agree, and in the instance of sound in health and healing, Laënnec's medico-sonic work in *de l'auscultation médiate* standardizes and shares—via rhetorical devices—sonic understandings of the body. Aided by the stethoscope, Laënnec could sonically amplify heart, intestine, and lung sounds. With *de l'auscultation médiate* and a stethoscope, other physicians could both read about and test Laënnec's similes and metaphors as they stand in for the body's heart, intestine, and lung sounds—the body's once ineffability and former onomatopoeia.

In the third edition of Forbes' translated version (1830), he gave this summary of *de l'auscultation médiate*:

From noting the sounds he [Laënnec] heard with his stethoscope during physical examinations of patients and linking them to pathological changes at post-mortem examination, Laënnec learned to recognise pulmonary diseases including bronchitis, bronchiectasis, emphysema, hydrothorax, pleurisy, pneumothorax, pneumonia, pulmonary gangrene, pulmonary oedema, and tuberculosis. Laënnec also came up with terms that are still in use—eg, bronchophony, egophony, and rales. *He described normal and abnormal sounds of respiration and different types of rales: crackling, crepitant, gurgling, sonorous, and whistling. Laënnec noted that pectoriloquy [resonance] was a sign indicating cavities in the lung caused by tuberculosis.*[49] (emphasis added)

Schafer pointed out that "the wind is an element that grasps the ears forcefully. The sensation is tactile as well as aural."[50] As air moves through our lungs, it can be heard. Laënnec capitalized on this certainty through auscultation, and he fashioned a system to clinically understand the body's sounds— whether aided by a stethoscope or not—to make sense of those sounds. Without getting waylaid in acoustics, sound is vibration that we can feel or hear (or do not—consider high-pitched whistles out of hearing human aural ranges). In addition to classifying heart, intestine, and lung sounds that he cross-referenced in autopsy findings, Laënnec also noted vibrations. Vibration is something we can feel, such as the reverberation of a hum in our throat—a tactile sensation—or the rumble of air through our bowels, which is also a tactile sensation. Sir Richard Paget, a trained physicist, theorized about the origin of language in his 1930 treatise on the ontology of spoken language, *Human Speech: Some Observations, Experiments, and Conclusions as to the Nature, Origin, Purpose and Possible Improvement of Human Speech*. In this work, Paget discussed the experiments he conducted, determining, "in recognizing speech sounds, the human ear is not listening to music but to indications, due to *resonance*, of the position and gestures of the organs of articulation"[51] (emphasis added), which I argue are also vibratory.

In his medico-sonic work, Laënnec accounted for vibration. For instance, he wrote, "there is also to be noticed a slight vibration communicated to the cylinder when the seat of the phenomenon happens to be immediately beneath it"[52]; and "the rhonchus [sound] is perceived over the whole sternum, and is accompanied by a vibration very perceptible to the touch: we can even sometimes perceive it over the whole chest and through the interposed lung."[53] To compare, Laënnec noted about normal breath, "Vhen [sic] a person in health speaks or sings, his voice excites in the whole walls of the thorax a sort of vibration, which is easily perceived on applying the hand to the chest."[54] Laënnec described abnormal breath sounds as

> This phenomenon is no longer observable, when, through disease, the lungs have ceased to be permeable to the air, or are removed from the walls of the chest by an effused fluid. This sign is, however, of inferior value, since a great many causes occasion varieties in the intensity of the vibration, or completely destroy it. For instance, it is little sensible in fat persons, in those whose integuments are rather flaccid, and in those who have a sharp and weak voice.[55]

Auenbrügger and Laënnec harnessed sound in two interrelated, yet different ways. Auenbrügger relied on percussion and its resultant tactilely sensed vibrations to make sense of the body, translating its sound to meld sonic understandings with cognitive, biomedical ones, creating his own medico-sonic understandings of the body through vibration and sound. Although Auenbrügger was not as successful as Laënnec at spreading this method of sonically amplifying the body—however rudimentary in comparison with contemporary biomedical efforts—ultimately, when paired together, percussion and auscultation amount to half of the currently practiced clinical methods used to biomedically and physically examine and assess people today. Laënnec credits the well-known Hippocrates for auscultation. However, there is evidence from translated texts that ancient physicians from Mesopotamia, Egypt, and India relied upon auscultation and percussion to assess and sonically account for sounds of disease in the body nearly 1,500 years before Hippocrates.

Mesopotamian Medicine, Cuneiform Script Translations, and Breath Sounds

Recorded examples reveal the body's sounds were used to make sense of disease over a millennium before Hippocrates. According to JoAnn Scurlock and Burton R. Andersen, "The oldest known ancient Mesopotamian medical text is a therapeutic manual, written in Sumerian, which dates from the Ur III period (2112–2004 B.C.E.)."[56] Written knowledge about the Mesopotamian practice of medicine both survives to the present and predates other ancient systems, which is how possibly one of the oldest available references to the use of sound in health and healing can be identified.[ii] Because the ancient Sumerian civilization of Mesopotamia devised cuneiform script into a writing system—one used for nearly 2,000 years throughout Mesopotamian city states (Assyria, Babylon, and Sumer)—several medical texts were preserved[57] that indicate that Mesopotamian medicine predates other ancient medical systems by over a millennia.

Even though Mesopotamian medicine was infused with supernatural and magical explanations of disease,[58] it also accounted for the importance of the pulmonary system, noting that "breathing and lung function were also known to be vital bodily activities that required prompt attention from the physician in the event of disease."[59] In Scurlock and Andersen's more recent translation, analysis, and synthesis of published and unpublished Mesopotamian cuneiform script medical texts titled *Diagnoses in Assyrian and Babylonian Medicine*, Andersen uses Scurlock's translations and descriptions to track onto modern Western biomedical knowledge. For example, in the chapter about the heart, circulatory system, and lungs Andersen describes asthma as "narrowed airways make it difficult to exhale, causing a high pitched wheezing sound ... that the patient can usually hear, and often can be heard at the patient's bedside without a stethoscope."[60] Scurlock and Andersen contend that "the physicians of ancient Mesopotamia were careful observers of clinical symptoms ... [and that] there is recorded evidence that physicians used all of their five senses except taste in observing their patients."[61] They listened to breath or lung[62] and bowel sounds.[63] The "lung sounds that are mentioned include wheezing, gurgling, growling noises, 'a mouth that roars,' gasping respiration, and deep breathing" or the "high-pitched expiratory noises found in asthma."[64] Scurlock and Andersen point out that it is unclear and unknown if these Mesopotamian physicians "listened to these breath sounds from the bedside, or actually put [their] ear to the patient's chest," yet reason that "the wheezing and gurgling sounds were noted by putting an ear to the patient's chest"[65] or through direct or immediate chest auscultation.

Scurlock translated several Sumerian script excerpts as containing such rhetorical devices as simile and metaphor. Examples include "gurgles like the waves of a canal," "so that his windpipe is full of wind," "he makes a loud growling noise," and "his lungs sing like a reed flute."[66] From Scurlock's translations and Andersen's descriptions, we can see that ancient attempts to reify medical understandings of the body included lung or breath sounds

ii For translations and analyses, see R. Campbell Thompson, *Assyrian Medical Texts: From the Originals in the British Museum* (London: Oxford University Press, 1923); Franz Köcher, ed., *Die babylonisch-assyrische Medizin in Texten und Untersuchungen* (Berlin: De Gruyter, 1963); and JoAnn Scurlock and Burton Andersen, *Diagnoses in Assyrian and Babylonian Medicine* (Champaign: University of Illinois Press, 2005).

compared with water ("waves"), wind, animal sounds ("growling"), and music ("reed flute"). Presumably, these similes and metaphors were used to make connections or draw comparisons among what physicians heard when immediately auscultating lungs for breath sounds and more commonly known, shared sounds. What is impressive is that it seems likely that the tablets containing this information—written in cuneiform script—also correlate sounds with pulmonary diseases, such as asthma[67] or even phthisis (or tuberculosis or other progressive pulmonary disease[68]).

Based on available evidence and translations, it also appears that attention to the body's sounds is not a one-off in ancient Mesopotamian medicine. The Codex Hammurapi or Hammurabi's Code—dated by experts from around 4,000 years ago—predates Hippocrates by more than a millennium.[69] In fact, one such preserved clay tablet translated from cuneiform script into English and from the seventh century BCE—*The Treatise of Medical Diagnosis and Prognosis*—mentions listening to a man's breath sounds and describing those sounds (attributed to tuberculosis) as "breathing [that] sounds like a flute."[70] The translation includes the rhetorical device simile ("like a flute") to describe breathing—another example of medico-sonic understandings mediated by rhetoric. From existing translations and what could be found, this Sumerian cuneiform script to English translation is likely one of the oldest mentions of what Western biomedicine would describe as breath sounds (or nonstethoscopic or immediate auscultation), and it is from the 17th century BCE. However, "the oldest surviving copy of this treatise dates to around 1600 BCE, [and] the information contained in the text is an amalgamation of several centuries of Mesopotamian medical knowledge,"[71] which makes the *Treatise* at least 3,600 years or nearly 4 millennia old, suggesting deeper, more ancient sonic roots than perhaps previously described or possibly acknowledged.

Egyptian Medicine, "debdeb," and Audible Signs of Disease

Hajar in "The Art of Listening" avers that "amongst the earliest known medical manuscripts are the medical papyruses of ancient Egypt dating to the 17th century BC, which referred to audible signs of disease within the body."[72] Living sometime between 2667 and 2648 BCE, the first physician known by name was Ihmotep, an Egyptian[73] (cf Herbowski[74]). In fact, some consider Ihmotep—not ancient Greek Hippocrates—to be the "true father" or founder of medicine or at least the eventual Egyptian patron of healers and medicine.[75] Ihmotep, called Imouthes (Greek: Ιμούθες), was held in regard alongside the Greek god of medicine, Aesclepius.[76] I point this out to redescribe common understandings about modern medicine and its roots and to argue that conventional, science-based allopathic or Western biomedical healthcare has possibly overlooked deeper, perhaps transcontinental (Africa and Asia), Egyptian roots.

What is known about ancient Egyptian medical practices survives via an extensive canon of ancient Egyptian papyri.[77] Of these hieratic papyri, translations of the Edwin Smith Papyrus (ESP) from the 17th century BCE and the Georg Ebers Papyrus (GEP) from the 16th century BCE are notable. These papyri provide descriptions of the Egyptian health system and their methods of clinical diagnosis. The ESP has even been thought to "quite obviously" be "a copy of a much older papyrus."[78] Although there's no way to be certain and any attempt to gain certainty is insuperable, it aligns with a theory that Ihmotep might have written the ESP originally.[79]

Ancient Egyptian medicine predates ancient Greek medicine by several millennia. In fact, in the introduction to the GEP, G. Elliott Smith noted that,

> it is often assumed even by the most learned historians that the history of medicine began with the Greeks, and that before the time of Hippocrates, there was little or nothing that could be called the science of medicine. Yet for more than thirty centuries before the emancipation of human reason in Ionia, numerous practitioners had been attempting to diagnose and treat disease in Egypt, Mesopotamia, and elsewhere.[80]

In fact, Ancient Egyptian medical practitioners relied upon listening to the body to identify "audible signs of disease" within it.[81] It has even been hypothesized in popular, web-based discourse that a medical instrument for listening is shown near the Wall of Twin Temple of Kom Ombo on the Nile (described as an ancient center for medical care in Egypt) (see Figure 2.3). Again, definitively knowing whether the object between what appears to be two cupping and scissor-like instruments depicts such a listening device is unknowable; however, the possibility remains.

Drawing upon evidence from French translations of GEP and English secondary sources like John F. Nunn's *Ancient Egyptian Medicine* that suggests that the Egyptians designated the sound of the heart as "debdeb,"[82] French physicians Bernard Ziskind and Bruno Halioua asked "*Les Égyptiens sont-ils les pionniers de l'auscultation?*"[83] ("Are Egyptians Pioneers of Auscultation?," written in French[iii]). Ziskind and Halioua support their hypothesis that Egyptian physicians listened to heart sounds by immediate auscultation by linking the auscultatory practice to *onomatopée*. They note that "The fact that the Egyptians used 'debdeb' to designate the beating of the heart may suggest it was through the ear and therefore through auscultation that they also examined the heart in the exercise of their art over 35 centuries ago."[84] They draw

---

iii I translated the original into English using a native French speaker's (Amélie Guyon) and a French-language learner's (Gustav Wiberg) advice and interpreted from comparing Google and Deep-L translated versions. I opted to use Deep-L translations. I appreciate and acknowledge their guidance.

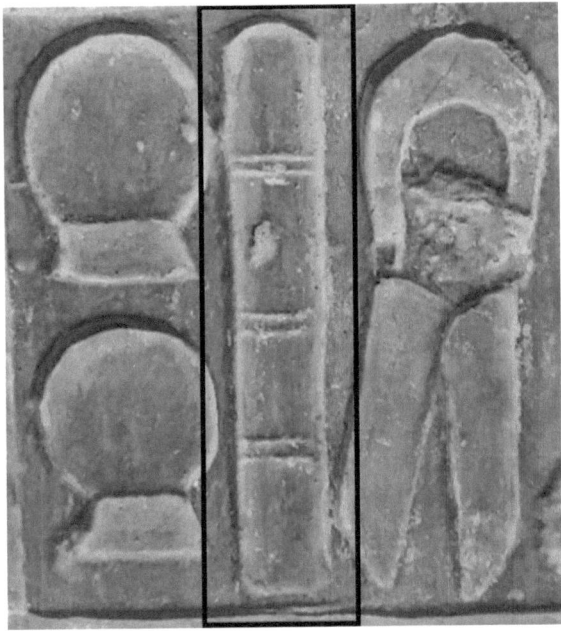

Figure 2.3 Photo of a replication of the Relief of Twin Temple of Kom Ombo on the Nile in Egypt. Medical instrumentation: two cupping devices (left), a long, perhaps listening instrument (middle), and shears (right) pictured; author photo.

comparisons from animals like cats referred to by their distinctive "miow (miw)" and lion "pronounced 'rou' (rw) by analogy to its roar"[85] to support their argument that Egyptians referred to sound, which at the very least makes logical and rhetorical sense.

Although palpation is known to be one ancient Egyptian physical examination method,[86,87] there is less evidence (available in existing translations of GEP) to account for auscultation or percussion as one. However, Ziskind and Halioua, relying on Thierry Bardinet's French translation of GEP directly from Egyptian hieratic in *Les Papyrus médicaux de l'Égypte pharaonique*,[88] use this excerpt from the Bardinet translation as basis for their hypothesis about Egyptian roots of auscultation (translated from French into English): "If you examine a man with an obstruction, his heart (inside -ib) trembles, his face is pale, his heart (inside -ib) makes debdeb noise (= pulsates)."[89] Some disagree with the "ib" translated as heart, instead suggesting it might mean all the internal organs other than the heart.[90] The "debdeb" as onomatopoeia and stand in for that which can't be put (at least easily) into words—or ineffable—is certainly rhetorically remarkable.

Unfortunately, auscultation and percussion as physical examination practices in translations of the ESP are not more definitively present or known. However, archaeologist James Henry Breasted[iv] noted that, along with palpation, "observation of the action of the heart by means of the pulse"[91] or what might be interpreted as ancient cardiac evaluation was practiced. As Breasted's former Egyptology student and scholar John A. Wilson described, ancient Egyptian physicians performed physical examinations, even if they did not specifically record what those physical processes entailed.[92] For example, the ESP reveals, "his heart beats feebly."[93] Wilson pointed out that both Ebers and Smith papyri "describe the beat of the heart as showing the condition of the patient"[94]; Wilson further contends that although "nothing is said about measuring the temperature of the body—presumably by palpation—about judging the condition of the eyes, tongue, or complexions ... these factors do appear as the examination is detailed in each case" presented in the ESP.[95]

What is to be done with translations of translations of hieratic script from so many millennia ago? It is reasonable to think Egyptian physicians relied on vibrations to take pulses and palpate their patients. It is a little less certain, although perhaps likely, that these ancient Egyptian physicians relied upon a physical examination process to ascertain audible signs of disease or understand the conditions of bodies they examined. However, whether by vibration and palpation or listening and immediate auscultation or percussion, ancient Egyptian physicians, given what we know about them today, likely understood more about allopathic—both observational and sonic—empirical ways of understanding the body, its injuries, conditions, and diseases than they are widely and explicitly given credit for. Ziskind and Halioua's onomatopoeiac "debdeb" signifies at the very least that ancient Egyptian physicians were close enough to bodies to identify an easily recognizable obstructed heart sound (the "debdeb"). This makes it likely that there was a normal heart sound the "debdeb" was compared with, and it mattered enough to be inscribed into papyrus. Their use of sound makes sense, as does the use of sound in ancient Mesopotamian medicine and in other ancient health and healing systems. The "debdeb" is an example of putting the ineffable into words. Or more accurately, rhetorical onomatopoeia into hieratic script. It also demonstrates that the onomatopoeia of the body's sounds—the formerly ineffable—were used to understand the body many millennia ago.

A Few Examples of Sound from Traditional Indian Medicine (Ayurveda)

With a more obvious case that demonstrates the use of sound in health and healing, take 5,000-year-old Ayurveda—traditional Indian medicine. Still

---

iv Editor-translator James Henry Breasted's 77-page "Special Introduction," reads like a rhetorical analysis of the ESP, including a careful categorization of the commentary and translation to come.

in practice and considered a CAM modality, ancient Ayurveda has listened for sounds to indicate health for several millennia. In addition to observing and questioning patients, Ayurveda practitioners use "listening for sounds made by the internal organs (Sanskrit: *shrvanaa*) and percussion or tapping (*akotana*)" to ascertain symptoms and determine treatments.[96] Physician Guido Majno relayed a description of Ayurvedic auscultation of an ulcer by Suśruta (Sanskrit: सुश्रुत)—the physician whose teachings contribute to the foundation of Ayurveda. In describing the Ayurvedic tradition, Majno explained that "most diseases were caused by deranged *vayu* or *vata*, the 'inner wind'; hence, in the words of Suśruta, '... a distinctively audible sound or report is heard in ... ulcers which are found charged with wind.'"[97] Majno continued, stating,

> The *vaidya* (physician) leaned over to sniff the cleaned-out ulcer at close quarters. Now the smell was just fishy, and therefore 'normal' for an ulcer. But what about the sound? He listened carefully, his ear to the ulcer. There was a definite sound of blowing, he said. The ulcer was charged with *vayu*, wind, that troublesome *dosha*[98] (italics added).

In an image that accompanies Majno's description of an Ayurvedic physician examining a foot ulcer, the Ayurvedic physician can be seen with their left hand cupping their left ear while immediately auscultating and listening for wind (*vayu*) of a foot ulcer wound.[99] The physician likely used their hand to cup their ear to amplify sound while listening to the wound. According to Kenneth G. Zysk in "The Science of Respiration and the Doctrine of the Bodily Winds in Ancient India," "Ancient Indians paid particular attention to respiration and the function of wind in the body by making the breathing process a focus of religious concern and practice."[100] For Ayurvedic medicine, the wind and breath are linked. The breath or *prāṇa* means "the breath in front," that is "the inhaled air."[101] *Prāṇa* (Sanskrit: प्राण) is Ayurvedically understood as coming from within the body, "and when expelled (through mouth or anus), produce[s] various sounds *resembling roars*"[102] (italics added). To contextualize Majno's explanation of the Ayurvedic physician auscultating the person's foot ulcer, Zysk explains that "the location of particular diseases in limbs or bodily parts is determined by the *faint sounds* connected to the limb or part and emitted by the patient"[103] (emphasis added).

Although my treatment of ancient Ayurvedic medicine and the role of immediate auscultation and *vayu* is not meant to be comprehensive, in this ancient medical system, auscultation or listening to the body was undertaken by physicians to understand ailments, afflictions, illness, and disease. *Vayu* or wind was listened for in ulcers via percussion (*akotana*) and the immediate auscultation (*shrvanaa*) of vital organs and body parts, such as in Majno's description. Even ancient Ayurvedic or Indian medical texts, like those Zysk analyzed and drew from in his examination of ancient bodily winds, use onomatopoeia for breath or *prāṇa* that when expelled resembled roars. When integrated with Ziskind and Halioua's hieratic translation of "rou" (rw) as roar[104] or Scurlock and Andersen's description of "a mouth that roars,"[105] animal-sound onomatopoeia is representative of bodily noises from ancient Mesopotamian, Egyptian, and Indian medicine. Although this might seem insignificant, in the context of sound in ancient health and healing contexts, rhetorically speaking onomatopoeia names the sound and attaches it to a known sound, which is a cognitive precursor to more rhetorically significant, medicosonic systematization through simile and metaphor—the sonic-cognitive building blocks of systematizing and sharing medico-sonic knowledge.

"Surely he ought to have added a fifth, that connected with hearing!": Ancient Greek and Roman Medicine

Even though ancient Greek physicians were influenced by other ancient (i.e., Egyptian, Cretan, and Babylonian) health systems and knowledge, medical writings from Egypt, India, and Mesopotamia are not known to be as widely circulated as those derived from Grecian medicine. For this reason, conventional, science-based, allopathic Western medicine's roots draw from ancient Greek medical knowledge.[106] Although I have presented examples of a possibility that the body's sounds from auscultation and percussion were used in ancient health and healing systems in Mesopotamia, Egypt, and India, most credit is given to the Greeks, particularly Hippocrates. For example, in an "Introductory Lecture to the Course on Materia Medica and Therapeutics" delivered at Guy's Hospital in central London and reprinted on May 16, 1874 in *BMJ*, W. Moxon mentioned Hippocrates on nearly every page and used Greek letters to draw connections from ancient Greek medicine to then current pharmacological or therapeutic content,[107] which possibly reveals a Euro-centric bias related to the foundation of medicine.

Although conventional, science-based, allopathic Western health systems are founded on his teachings, not much is reliably known about Hippocrates himself.[108] Majno in *The Healing Hand* claimed that "after Hippocrates, auscultation was forgotten."[109] However, in addition to his fluency in Latin and Greek,[110] Laënnec studied the writings of Hippocrates and composed his doctor of medicine thesis about him in "*Propositions sur la doctrine d'Hippocrate appliqué à la medicine-pratique.*"[111] Greek physicians used direct, or immediate, auscultation to physically assess their patients. Forbes noted that

according to the expression of M. Bayle, to be no less skilled in the knowledge of the Greek language than deeply read in the writings of the father of physic [sic]. M. Laënnec was, indeed, always a great admirer of Hyppocrates [sic]; and there are few of his writings in which this admiration is not strongly expressed.[112]

In *de l'auscultation médiate*, Laënnec—through Forbes's translation—wrote:

> I ought to be the less surprised at these unsuccessful results of my attempts, as Hippocrates himself, as I have elsewhere shown, committed the same mistake. But if auscultation by itself and not, as Hippocrates supposed, detect the presence of a fluid in the chest, we obtain at least from the writings of this great man, or those of his disciples, a sign very characteristic of this affection, in one particular form of it.[113]

There are over 60 treatises in the *Hippocratic Corpus* that are sometimes attributed to him, including methods to physically diagnose patients. Of note, Hippocrates recommended a procedure resembling "direct"[114] or immediate auscultation—the method of applying the ear directly to the chest—that involved "shaking a patient by the shoulders—succussion—and listening for sounds evoked by the chest … in order to detect the accumulation of fluid within the chest."[115] Laënnec was familiar with Hippocrates's auscultation-like practice of succussion or the Hippocratic succussion splash described as hydropneumothorax—the presence of air and fluid in the lungs.[116]

Laënnec described succussion as follows:

> This method of exploration, which perhaps has never been practised but by the Asclepiades [of Bithynia], consists in shaking the patient's trunk, and at the same time listening to the sounds thereby produced. This process is described by the author of the treatise *De Morbis* (lib. ii. 45) in the following terms: "Having placed the patient in a firm seat, cause his hands to be held by an assistant, and then shake him by the shoulder, in order to hear on which side the disease shall produce a sound."[117]

Although Hippocrates is credited as the originating physician of immediate auscultation in various scientific and scholarly sources,[118] there is no certainty in that assertion, and it seems Hippocrates did not systematically explore body sounds and meanings through immediate auscultation.[119] In fact, physician and medical historian Stanley Joel Reiser asserted in *Medicine and the Reign of Technology* that

> Hippocrates was the first to describe the basic aspect of auscultation in *De Morbis*: "You shall know by this that the chest contains water and not pus, if in applying the ear during a certain time on the side, you perceive a noise like that of boiling vinegar."[120]

Popularization credit likely belongs—like the Auenbrügger–Corvisart–Laënnec percussion-auscultation influence—to other ancient physicians, such as those from ancient Egypt, Crete, or Mesopotamia (standing on or rather listening from the shoulders of giants and such). Essentially, it seems likely that sound was used to physically assess bodies in ancient Greece and later—and somewhat more recently—in ancient Rome.

What is notable in the Reiser explanation that draws from the same text Laënnec[121] references—*De Morbis*—is the comparison of the lung sound to "a noise like that of boiling vinegar," which Majno also writes about "as if it were boiling inside like vinegar."[122] As a rhetorical device here, the simile stands in for the ineffable—the lung sound itself—and draws a comparison to what might have been a sound other physicians would know. To test this comparison, Majno heated, then boiled vinegar and noted it sounded like "rushing, crackling noise, quite unlike that of boiling water, and comparing very well with the sound heard over a lung when fluid obstructs the finest bronchi, a sound called 'a fine moist rales' in modern terminology."[123] Majno reasoned that ancient Greek physicians would likely be familiar with a boiling vinegar sound because boiling vinegar was "a common step in preparing drugs and plasters," which was part of their work.[124] Majno's explanation makes sense, especially since when similes and metaphors are successfully used, they rely on (the physician's) familiarity with the comparison. To better understand the comparison, I boiled vinegar, which did indeed rush and crack and pop—it sounded distinctive from boiling water.

It seems that modern physician-translators accept Hippocrates practiced and taught auscultation (even if scholars of the history of medicine do not and contest whether Hippocrates wrote any of the works commonly attributed to him[125]). From a summary compilation epitomized by translator John Redman Coxe (1846),[126] *The Writings of Hippocrates and Galen*, Coxe uses the original Latin (Albrecht von Haller selected and compiled existing Latin translations[127] in 1775) from *De Morbis*, "*Tu vero agitato humero, quonam in latere (affectio) streptitum edat, auscultato.*"[128] Recall that *ausculto* means "to listen," which orients an understanding of Coxe's Latin-English translation: "Auscultation is here clearly adverted [sic] to, and incision ordered for the removal of the pus."[129] Less definitive references in Coxe's summary of *De Morbis* noted that "something like auscultation alluded to,"[130] "auscultation is obviously spoken of,"[131] and "auscultation apparently adverted [sic] to"[132] in pulmonary contexts, such as the thorax or chest in the two former; dropsy or edema and lungs in the latter.

In a section on aphorisms in *Hippocratic Writings*, Geoffrey Ernest Richard Lloyd identified "respiration characterized by a sobbing sound in acute febrile illnesses is a bad sign,"[133] and "sneezing occurs when the brain becomes thoroughly heated or when the sinuses become thoroughly moistened or chilled. As a result, the air within is pushed out … makes a noise because its exit is through a narrow passage."[134] A treatise translation of *On Ancient Medicine* in Lloyd's volume (described as "an explanation of the empirical basis of medicine as practised about the end of the fifth century [CE]"[135]) noted that

> the organs of the body that cause flatulence and colic, such as the stomach and chest, produce noise and rumbling. For any hollow organ that does not become full of fluid and remain [sic] so but instead undergoes changes and movement, must necessarily produce noises and the signs of movement.[136]

From Lloyd's explanation, it appears that the body in ancient Greece was sonically attended to by physicians (whether Hippocrates did or not). And, from other sources, it seems percussion was used as a remedy to the problem of ancient and erroneous conceptions about the wandering womb.[137] Christopher A. Faraone compiled Greek antiquarian medical knowledge about the wandering womb or uterus in "Magical and Medical Approaches to the Wandering Womb in the Ancient Greek World," noting that when it "shifts out of place," percussion was one of several treatments used by ancient Greek physicians.[138] Again, the sometimes dubious considerations of translations across language, culture, and time aside, these references—these scattered sonic fragments of understanding the sounds of the body—suggest that sound was employed to understand the body, perhaps even though unnamed, through ancient versions of auscultation and percussion.

Since ancient Romans were unable to be physicians,[139] at this intersection of sonic treatments for ancient Greek roving uteri, it is apt to introduce Galen. He was educated in both philosophy and rhetoric and practiced medicine as a Greek physician in Rome in the first century of the Common Era (CE) or about 2,000 years ago. The Greek influence on Roman medicine is well-documented and logical because

> in Rome, ... physicians were looked upon as a different breed of creature. For one thing, most of them were Greeks. Tradition forbade that Romans themselves practice medicine. Just like other artistic talents, such as that for music, dance, poetry, magic, etc, medicine was considered a profession 'worthy only for slaves, freedmen, or foreigners' who were, of course, Greeks![140]

In the 700 treatises and writings attributed to Galen and summarized in Coxe's *The Writings of Hippocrates and Galen*, we next look to the sixth volume *De Differentiis Morborum Et Causis, Symptomatumque*, or "Of the Differences and Causes of Diseases and Symptoms."[141] In the book about the difference of symptoms or *De Symptomatum Differentiis* (Book III), Coxe states

> Galen says something as to the five senses, and points out the symptoms arising from their diseased action. Symptoms are said to be of a fourfold

nature; some are visible, some sensible to the smell, some to the taste, and some to the touch. *Surely he ought to have added a fifth, that connected with hearing!*[142,v] (italics added)

Hippocrates is widely, if not perhaps erroneously, thought to have used direct auscultation and taught it as a method to students. It seems apparent that Majno's assertion from *The Healing Hand* is likely. And since Hippocrates's auscultation slipped out of use,[143] it echoes as probable from across these ancient civilizations and over the past two millennia. In this instance rhetorical pan-historiography reveals a range of "miniature studies"[144] of rhetoric and sound in health and healing across ancient health and healing systems with "each making its own point that contributes to, even as it [potentially] complicates, the longer view."[145] With a pan-historiographic approach, I demonstrate what a sonic lineage for sound in health and healing might look like when mediated by rhetoric—perhaps revealing an opening for Auenbrügger's work on percussion and Laënnec's resurrection of immediate auscultation.

The entirety of this chapter explicitly answers how sound was used in ancient and CAM health and healing systems. From what we can accurately know based on recorded, preserved, and translated history, whether cuneiform or hieratic script or written in any known or modern language and from his own writings, there is an ancient rhetorical foundation from Mesopotamia, Egypt, and India for Hippocrates and at least his contemporaries and Galen and later Corvisart and Auenbrügger to build upon. Each influenced—Hippocrates and Auenbrügger especially and explicitly—Laënnec's thinking about sound and its use in health and healing.

The use of rhetorical devices, such as onomatopoeia, simile, and metaphor, also supported and enabled sonic understandings of the body in ancient health and healing systems. An answer to "How does ineffable bodily sound in health and healing use rhetoric to transform?" is demonstrated simply by "debdeb" and transforming bodily sounds into written and spoken language via onomatopoeia. Without rhetoric, the body's sounds are not understandable, knowable, or treatable. Without onomatopoeia, a sonic lexicon for bodily sounds could not be known for an incomparable historical-cultural moment to come millennia later: Laënnec's medico-sonic work, which—as I argue—relies on and builds upon an interplay between rhetoric and sound. Without Laënnec's medico-sonic work, science-based, allopathic Western biomedicine would not exist as we know it. Powered by rhetoric, Laënnec's medico-sonic work contributed to harnessing sound for diagnostic, prognostic, and therapeutic methods, which act as rhetorical ventriloquists as I show in Chapter 4.

---

v   Armed with two years of high school Latin, one year of university Spanish, three courses in Swedish, and one course in workplace German, after wading through translations of millennia-old works spanning hundreds of years and multiple languages, I wholeheartedly agree.

Notes

1 Shannon Mattern, "Urban Auscultation; or, Perceiving the Action of the Heart," *Places* (April 2020): para. 6. https://placesjournal.org/article/urban-auscultation-or-perceiving-the-action-of-the-heart/?cn-reloaded=1

2 Guido Majno, *The Healing Hand: Man and Wound in the Ancient World* (Cambridge, MA: Harvard University Press, 1991), 170.

3 Walker, *Clinical Methods*, 5.

4 Gregory Tscoucalas and Markos Sgantzos, "Hippocrates, on the Infection of the Lower Respiratory Tract among the General Population in Ancient Greece," *General Medicine: Open Access* 4, no. 5 (2016): 2. https://doi.org/10.4172/2327-5146.1000272.

5 René Theophile-Hyacinthe Laënnec, *A Treatise on the Diseases of the Chest and on Mediate Auscultation*, trans. John Forbes (New York: Samuel Wood & Sons, 1838), 347, https://collections.nlm.nih.gov/ext/mhl/9308216/PDF/9308216.pdf.

6 Jenny Edbauer, "Unframing Models of Public Distribution: From Rhetorical Situation to Rhetorical Ecologies," *Rhetoric Society Quarterly* 35, no. 4 (2005): 20. https://repositories.lib.utexas.edu/bitstream/handle/2152/1541/edbauerj59267.pdf.

7 Debra Hawhee and Christa J. Olson, "Pan-historiography: The Challenges of Writing History across Time and Space," in *Theorizing Histories of Rhetoric* (Carbondale, IL: Southern Illinois University Press, 2013), 90–105.

8 Rachel Hajar, "The Art of Listening," *Heart Views* 13, no. 1 (January–March 2012): 24, https://doi.org/10.4103/1995-705X.96668.

9 Lippincott Williams & Wilkins, Inc. "Assessing Patients Effectively: Here's How to Do the Basic Four Techniques," *Nursing* 8, no. 2 (November 2006): 6, https://journals.lww.com/nursing/Fulltext/2006/11002/Assessing_patients_effectively__Here_s_how_to_do.5.aspx.

10 Tom Rice, "Learning to Listen: Auscultation and the Transmission of Auditory Knowledge," *Journal of the Royal Anthropological Institute* 16 (2010): S41, http://www.jstor.org/stable/40606064.

11 "Assessing Patients Effectively," 6.

12 "Percussion," Medline Plus, U.S. National Library of Medicine, https://medlineplus.gov/ency/article/002226.htm.

13 "Assessing Patients Effectively," 6.

14 Ibid., para. 2.

15 Ibid., para. 3.

16 Ibid., para. 3.

17 "Assessing Patients Effectively," 6.

18 Rice, "Learning to Listen," S41.

19 "Assessing Patients Effectively," 6.

20 Austin Flint and J.C. Wilson, *A Manual Auscultation and Percussion: Embracing the Physical Diagnosis of Diseases of the Lungs and Heart, and of Thoracic Aneurism* (1890). Flickr, 10 January 2024. https://www.flickr.com/photos/internetarchivebookimages/14748163536/in/photolist-odNptR-otfccE-ox2Yhi-ovfq7w-ovh8mX-odMzrE-otfdu9-odNqzD-odMzD3-otfbNo-ouZTFD-odMvSM-odNoMa./

21 Rice, "Learning to Listen."

22 Ibid., S42–S43.

23 Noreen Iftikhar, "What is Allopathic Medicine?" *Healthline*, last reviewed on May 28, 2019, https://www.healthline.com/health/allopathic-medicine

24 Hawhee and Olson, "Pan-historiography," 103.

25 Ibid., 103.

26 J. James Smith, "The *Inventum Novum* of Joseph Leopold Auenbrügger," *Bulletin of the New York Academy of Medicine* 38, no. 10 (1962), 696; H. Kenneth Walker, W. D. Hall, and J. W. Hurst, eds., *Clinical Methods: The History, Physical, and Laboratory Examinations,* 3rd ed. (Boston: Butterworths, 1990), 10.
27 Walker, *Clinical Methods*, 5.
28 Hajar, "The Art of Listening," 24.
29 Alex Sakula, "R. T. H. Laënnec 1781–1826 His Life and Work: A Bicentenary Appreciation," *Thorax* 36, no. 2 (1981): 84, http://dx.doi.org/10.1136/thx.36.2.81.
30 Walker, *Clinical Methods*, 10.
31 Ibid.
32 Smith, "The *Inventum Novum*."
33 Forbes, "A Treatise on the Diseases," 15–16.
34 Hajar, "The Art of Listening," 24.
35 Mark Pottinger, "Lucia and the Auscultation of Disease in Mid-Nineteenth-Century France," *Nineteenth-Century Music Review* 1–30 (2020). https://doi.org/10.1017/S1479409820000075.
36 Forbes, "A Treatise on the Diseases," 11.
37 Sakula, "R. T. H. Laënnec," 84.
38 Farhat Yaqub, "René Théophile Hyachinthe Laënnec," *Lancet Respiratory Medicine* 3, no. 10 (2015): 755, https://doi.org/10.1016/S2213-2600(15)00374-4.
39 Sakula, "R. T. H. Laënnec," 82.
40 Ibid., 83.
41 Yaqub, "René Théophile Hyachinthe Laënnec," 755.
42 Forbes, "A Treatise on the Diseases," xxii.
43 Sakula, "R. T. H. Laënnec," 81.
44 Yaqub, "René Théophile Hyachinthe Laënnec," 756.
45 Forbes, "A Treatise on the Diseases," 566.
46 Ibid., 556.
47 Ibid., 566.
48 Jonathan Sterne, ed., *The Sound Studies Reader* (New York: Routledge, 2012), 8, https://ia800308.us.archive.org/10/items/orejainculta-antropologia-sonora/14. Sterne_the%20sound%20studies%20reader.pdf.
49 Yaqub, "René Théophile Hyachinthe Laënnec," 756.
50 F. Murray Schafer, *The Soundscape: Our Sonic Environment and the Tuning of the World* (Rochester, VT: Destiny Books, 1977/1994), 22.
51 Richard Paget, *Human Speech: Some Observations, Experiments, and Conclusions as to the Nature, Origin, Purpose and Possible Improvement of Human Speech* (London: Kegan Paul, Ltd. and Routledge, 1930), 125.
52 Forbes, "A Treatise on the Diseases," 57.
53 Ibid., 11.
54 Ibid., 10.
55 Ibid., 10.
56 JoAnn Scurlock and Burton Andersen, *Diagnoses in Assyrian and Babylonian Medicine* (Champaign: University of Illinois Press, 2005), 25.
57 Lyn Robinson, *Understanding Healthcare Information* (London: Facet Publishing, 2010), 40.
58 Allen D. Spiegel and Christopher R. Springer, "Babylonian Medicine, Managed Care and Codex Hammurabi, Circa 1700 B.C.," *Journal of Community Health* 22, no. 1 (1997): 74.
59 Scurlock and Andersen, *Diagnoses in Assyrian and Babylonian Medicine*, 184.
60 Ibid.
61 Ibid., 8.
62 Ibid., 180.

63 Ibid., 2.
64 Ibid., 180.
65 Ibid., 180.
66 Ibid., 181, 184.
67 Ibid., 184.
68 Spiegel and Springer, "Babylonian Medicine," 74.
69 Ibid., 69.
70 Roy Porter, *The Greatest Benefit to Mankind: A Medical History of Humanity* (New York: W. W. Norton & Co., 1997), 45.
71 "The Largest Surviving Medical Treatise from Ancient Mesopotamia," Jeremy Norman's HistoryofInformation.com, https://www.historyofinformation.com/detail.php?id=2155.
72 Hajar, "The Art of Listening," 24.
73 Zelimir Mikić, "Imhotep—Builder, Physician, God," *Medicinski pregled* (Serbia) 61, no. 9–10 (September–October 2008): para. 1.
74 Leszek Herbowski. "The Maze of the Cerebrospinal Fluid Discovery." *Anatomy Research International*, 596027 (2013).
75 "Imhotep, Active 2667 B.C.–2648 B.C.," Library of Congress, http://id.loc.gov/authorities/names/no2005090540
76 Mikić, "Imhotep—Builder, Physician, God," para. 3.
77 Alexander Brawanski, "On the Myth of the Edwin Smith Papyrus: Is It Magic or Science?," *Acta Neurochirugica* 154, no. 12 (2012): 2285).
78 Brawanski, "On the Myth of the Edwin Smith Papyrus," 2285; Cyril P. Bryan, trans., *Ancient Egyptian Medicine: The Papyrus Ebers* (Chicago, IL: Ares Publishers Inc., 1930): xiv.
79 Mikić, "Imhotep—Builder, Physician, God," para. 3.
80 Bryan, *Ancient Egyptian Medicine*, xiii.
81 Hajar, "The Art of Listening," 24.
82 J. F. Nunn, Review of *Les Papyrus médicaux de l'Égypte pharaonique*, by Thierry Bardinet, *Medical History* 40, no. 2 (April 1996).
83 Bernard Ziskind and Bruno Halioua, "Les Égyptiens sont-ils les pionniers de l'auscultation?," *La Presse Médicale* 32, no. 32 (2003): 1507.
84 Ziskind and Halioua, "Les Égyptiens," 1507. DeepL Translation.
85 Ziskind and Halioua, "Les Égyptiens," 1507.
86 See Cyril P. Bryan, trans., *Ancient Egyptian Medicine: The Papyrus Ebers* (Chicago, IL: Ares Publishers, Inc., 1930), 129.
87 James Henry Breasted, ed., trans., *The Edwin Smith Surgical Papyrus: published in facsimile and hieroglyphic transliteration with translation and commentary in two volumes*," vol. 1 (Chicago, IL: The University of Chicago Oriental Institute Publications, 1930), 7.
88 Thierry Bardinet, *Les Papyrus médicaux de l'Égypte pharaonique* (Paris: Fayard, 1995).
89 As cited in Ziskind and Halioua, "Les Égyptiens," 1507.
90 Nunn, Review of *Les Papyrus médicaux*.
91 Breasted, p. 7
92 John A. Wilson, "Medicine in Ancient Egypt," *Bulletin of the History of Medicine* 36, no. 2 (March–April 1962): 114–23, https://www.jstor.org/stable/44449784?seq=1.
93 (Breasted, p. 177).
94 Ibid., 116.
95 Ibid., 121.
96 Amala Guha, "What Happens in a Visit to an Ayurvedic Practitioner?," Taking Charge of your Health & Wellbeing, para. 3–5, https://www.takingcharge.csh.umn.edu/explore-healing-practices/ayurvedic-medicine/what-happens-visit-ayurvedic-practitioner.

97 Majno, *The Healing Hand,* 299.
98 Ibid.
99 Majno, *The Healing Hand,* 299.
100 Kenny G. Zysk, "The Science of Respiration and the Doctrine of the Bodily Winds in Ancient India," *Journal of the American Oriental Society* 113, no, 2 (1993): 198.
101 Ibid., 198.
102 Ibid., 204.
103 Ibid., 212.
104 Ziskind and Halioua, "Les Égyptiens," 1507.
105 Scurlock and Andersen, *Diagnoses in Assyrian and Babylonian Medicine,* 180.
106 Walker, *Clinical Methods,* 5.
107 W. Moxon, "Introductory Lecture to the Course on Materia Medica and Therapeutics Delivered at Guy's Hospital," *British Medical Journal* 1, no. 698 (May 16, 1874): 635–40.
108 Christos Yapijakis, "Hippocrates of Kos, the Father of Clinical Medicine, and Asclepiades of Bithynia, the Father of Molecular Medicine," *In Vivo* 23, no. 4 (July 2009): 507–14.
109 Majno, *The Healing Hand,* 492.
110 Sakula, "R. T. H. Laënnec."
111 Forbes, "A Treatise on the Diseases," xvi.
112 Ibid.
113 Ibid., 539.
114 Walker, *Clinical Methods,* 5.
115 Hajar, "The Art of Listening," 24.
116 Geetha Girithari, Inês Coelho dos Santos, Eva Claro, Serguey Belykh, David Matias, and Orlando Santos. "The Hippocratic Splash," *European Journal of Case Reports in Internal Medicine* 5, no. 11 (2018): 000975, para. 5, https://doi.org/10.12890/2018_000975.
117 Forbes, "A Treatise on the Diseases," 539.
118 Walker, *Clinical Methods*; Forbes, "A Treatise on the Diseases"; Girithari et al., "The Hippocratic Splash."
119 Stanley Joel Reiser, *Medicine and the Reign of Technology* (Cambridge: Cambridge University Press, 1981), 24.
120 Reiser, *Medicine and the Reign of Technology,* 23.
121 Forbes, trans., "A Treatise on the Diseases of the Chest and on Mediate Auscultation," 28–29.
122 Majno, *The Healing Hand,* 170.
123 Ibid., 171.
124 Ibid.
125 Hubert Steinke, email message to author, January 11, 2022. Steinke is a physician, an Albrecht von Haller scholar, and a scholar of the history of medicine at the University of Bern, Switzerland, Institute for the History of Medicine.
126 Ibid.
127 Ibid.
128 John Redman Coxe, *The Writings of Hippocrates and Galen: Epitomised from the Original Latin Translations* (Philadelphia: Lindsay and Blakiston, 1846), https://oll-resources.s3.us-east-2.amazonaws.com/oll3/store/titles/1988/HippocratesGalen_0881_EBk_v6.0.pdf.
129 Ibid., 196.
130 Ibid., 200.
131 Ibid., 201.
132 Ibid., 210.

133 G. E. R. Lloyd, ed., *Hippocratic Writings* (London: Penguin Books, 1983), 230.
134 Lloyd, *Hippocratic Writings*, 234.
135 Ibid., 70.
136 Ibid., 85.
137 See Amy Koerber, *From Hysteria to Hormones: A Rhetorical History* (University Park: Pennsylvania State University Press, 2018), vol. 7.
138 Christopher A. Faraone, "Magical and Medical Approaches to the Wandering Womb in the Ancient Greek World," *Classical Antiquity* 30, no. 1 (April 2011), 24.
139 T. N. K. Raju, "Soranus of Ephesus: Who Was He and What Did He Do?" in *Historical Review and Recent Advances in Neonatal and Perinatal Medicine*, eds. George F. Smith and Dharmapuri Vidyasagar (Chicago, IL: Mead Johnson Nutritional Division, 1980), para. 6.
140 A. Castaglioni, *A History of Medicine*. (New York: Alfred-Knopf, 1941), 149–751; Raju, "Soranus of Ephesus," para. 6.
141 *Complectens, cui insunt quæ de morborum ac symptomatum causis differentiisque; et reliqua hisce finitima materia per artem totam traduntur, unà cum commentariis in libros Hippocratis, de morbis vulgaribus*, Basil Edition, 1549, 6. Retrieved from https://oll-resources.s3.us-east-2.amazonaws.com/oll3/store/titles/1988/HippocratesGalen_0881_EBk_v6.0.pdf
142 Coxe, *The Writings of Hippocrates and Galen*, 440.
143 Majno, *The Healing Hand*, 492.
144 Hawhee and Olson, "Pan-historiography," 98.
145 Hawhee and Olson, "Pan-historiography," 98.

3 Integrating Rhetoric with the Sonic and the Body

Intentional and Unintentional
Diagnostic, Prognostic, and
Therapeutic Uses of Sound
in Contemporary Western
Biomedical Health Systems

Ancient, enduring methods to understand the body using sound relied on rhetoric and a figure of sound—onomatopoeia—to do so. In the previous chapter, I used Debra Hawhee and Christa J. Olson's methodology pan-historiography[1] to trace the body's sounds. I also rhetorically presented scattered, translated examples of auscultation and percussion in ancient health systems as clinical interpretation of "audible signs of disease within the body"[2] by naked and likely unaided ears. I argued for the transformation of knowledge about the body's ineffability as onomatopoeia using rhetorical devices. Rhetorical devices metaphor and simile gradually enabled the once ineffable to further transform from onomatopoeia into a codified medico-sonic system of knowledge to understand the body. From making meaning with the sonic qualities of our bodies and making our bodies sonic, it led to cataloguing and deploying sonic knowledge about bodies in medical education and training. Laënnec's 1819 work *de l'auscultation mediate* eventually harnessed a rhetoric-sonic interplay, which noticeably emerges as rhetorically-powered medico-sonic knowledge.

Sound and listening to the body are part of its ancient allopathic[3] lineage—one that I used pan-historiography to redescribe as rhetorical in Chapter 2. The rhetorical transformation of sound traced in the previous chapter interpreted "audible signs of disease within the body"[4] with naked and unaided ears from scattered, yet contiguous instances of auscultation and percussion in ancient health systems. I further demonstrate a rhetoric-sonic interplay as integral for enabling sound's use in health and healing. I again draw from Hawhee and Olson's pan-historiography by continuing a diachronic approach examining the interplay of sound and rhetoric "across geographic space, tracking important ... practices as they travel ...."[5] Ultimately, sound in health and healing draws, yields, and fortifies persuasive, rhetorical power when deployed medically and intentionally through diagnostic, prognostic, and therapeutic uses of sound in health and healing. Rhetorically powered sound also boosts

DOI: 10.4324/9781032724416-3

unintentional, non-medical uses of sound—an argument developed in the next chapter. More modern integrations of the body with healthcare technologies rely on sound reproduction, such as physiological monitors or ultrasound; however, I argue Laënnec's *de l'auscultation mediate* and its medico-sonic content are the foundation for using sound diagnostically, prognostically, and therapeutically in conventional, science-based allopathic Western biomedical care—an argument hinging on a rhetoric-sonic interplay and Laënnec's invention of the stethoscope.

A Quire of Paper: The Origin of the Stethoscope

The stethoscope (Figure 3.1) is a recognizable symbol worn by members of various health professions, such as physician, nurse, and respiratory therapist. It is a symbol "giv[ing] presence, meaning, and value to a technological object or process within a discursive system."[6] A stethoscope is an acoustical medical device used for mediate auscultation, which derives from the Greek *stethos* (chest) and *skopein* (to look at or to observe). The stethoscope is also a teleological medical artifact—its purpose explains its design; its design explains its purpose. It cognitively gathers and orients collected knowledge over time for immediate application—like Edwin Hutchin's astrolabe for Polynesian navigators[7]; the knowledge is temporally distributed, culturally situated, and medico-sonic across several millennia. In a Tweet by Chicago's International Museum of Surgical Science, the stethoscope was identified as a

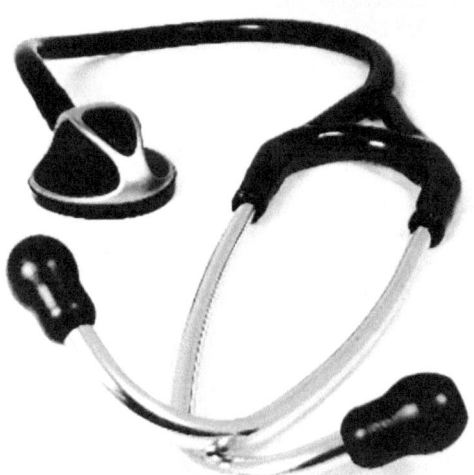

Figure 3.1 The modern stethoscope—a symbol of health workers everywhere.[9]

medical instrument designed by Laënnec in 1816 to avoid "press[ing] ... ears directly against a patient's chest to hear their lungs!"[8]

Included at length in his own words and translated by Forbes, Laënnec recounted the stethoscope's purpose and described his invention as being prompted when,

> In 1816, I was consulted by a young woman labouring under general symptoms of diseased heart, and in whose case percussion and the application of the hand were of little avail on account of the great degree of fatness. The other method just mentioned being rendered inadmissible by the age and sex of the patient, I happened to recollect a simple and well-known fact in acoustics, and fancied it might be turned to some use on the present occasion. The fact I allude to is the great distinctness with which we hear the scratch of a pin at one end of a piece of wood, on applying our ear to the other. Immediately, on this suggestion, I rolled a quire of paper into a kind of cylinder and applied one end of it to the region of the heart and the other to my ear, and was not a little surprised and pleased, to find that I could thereby perceive the action of the heart in a manner much more clear and distinct than I had ever been able to do by the immediate application of the ear. From this moment I imagined that the circumstance might furnish means for enabling us to ascertain the character, not only of the action of the heart, but of every species of sound produced by the motion of all the thoracic viscera, and, consequently, for the exploration of the respiration, the voice, the rhonchus, and perhaps even the fluctuation of fluid extravasated in the pleura or the pericardium. With this conviction, I forthwith commenced at the Hospital Necker [in Paris] a series of observations from which I have been able to deduce *a set of new signs of diseases of the chest, for the most part certain, simple, and prominent, and calculated, perhaps, to render the diagnosis of the diseases of the lungs, heart, and pleura, as decided and circumstantial*, as the indications furnished to the surgeon by the introduction of the finger or sound, in the complaints wherein these are used.[10]

Rhetorical ecology acts as a frame for understanding Laënnec's description of the events. Edbauer offers affective ecologies that "recontextualize[d] rhetorics in their temporal, historical, and lived fluxes ... as a circulating ecology of effects, enactments, and events by shifting the lines of focus from rhetorical situation to rhetorical ecologies."[11] Laënnec describes the events that led to the exigency for his invention (i.e., immediate auscultation failing to reveal a patient's heart sounds) and prompted his drawing upon acoustical knowledge (i.e., "recollect[ing] a simple and well-known fact in acoustics") to create the first stethoscope out of paper (i.e., rolling paper into a cylinder aimed to amplify a sound for the listener). The description is remarkable because he reveals an awareness of what the stethoscope can do for the physician by attending to the sounds and noises of the body—"the lived, in-process operations of this rhetoric"[12] and how the sounds represent "a set of new signs of diseases of the chest."

Laënnec's use of rhetoric is also a material feminist one. In their collection, Alaimo and Hekman bring together scholarship examining the "materiality of the human body and the natural world"—the once discarded, new material feminist approach they endorse.[13] The distributed sonic knowledge is an "evolving corporeal practice[e]"[14] embedded into the stethoscope. From the body's ineffability to the onomatopoeia of the ancient Egyptian hieratic "debdeb"; through similes and metaphors that stand in for onomatopoeia in Hippocratic descriptions; to Laënnec's development and inscription of medico-sonic knowledge in *de l'auscultation médiate*; the knowledge about the body's sounds accreted and waxed and waned over time. The knowledge demonstrates an evolving corporeal practice. For example, Laënnec stated that "every species of sound produced by the motion of all the thoracic viscera [chest], and, consequently, for the exploration of the respiration [lungs], the voice, *the rhonchus* [sound], and perhaps even the fluctuation of fluid extravasated in the pleura [lungs] or the pericardium [heart]"[15] (emphasis original) produced sonic or auditory signs he categorized and inscribed with rhetoric and as rhetorical devices in *de l'auscultation médiate*.

Later, Laënnec wrote,

When I first began to make use of the stethoscope, I was in hopes that this instrument might furnish some sign, analogous to the rhonchus [sound], calculated to discover collections of serum or pus within the chest, by means of fluctuation. Two methods of effecting this exploration naturally presented themselves: one was to percuss the chest on one side, as in ascites, and apply the stethoscope to the opposite one; the other was to listen simply to the sounds occasioned by the agitation of the fluid from the natural action of the heart and lungs.[16]

As a medical artifact and tool, the stethoscope is over 200 years old. However, wireless Bluetooth stethoscopes for deaf users are newer technologies. TikTok creator and medical student Alexandra Elaine—the United Kingdom's "first deafblind person training to be a Doctor [sic; physician]" explains how she uses a wireless Bluetooth stethoscope that connects to her hearing aids for "super hearing"; she further explains that she is "profoundly deaf"[17] and without her hearing aids, she is in "total silence," yet with her hearing aids, she can "hear enough" for a "face[-to]-face" conversation through "a mixture of sound vibrations, vowel sounds, and common sense."[18] The stethoscope she uses is a Thinklabs One digital stethoscope, which amplifies sound over one hundred times and connects to audio headphones, or for Alexandra Elaine's hearing aids, to amplify sound: "the loudest stethoscope ever made [… with] fully adjustable volume (1–10) to fit the audio needs of any individual."[19]

When used as an assistive technology for deaf healthcare clinicians or people with hearing disabilities, digital stethoscopes amplify the body's sounds and provide acoustic clinical information.

Hopeful conjecture about an ancient Egyptian tool like a stethoscope aside (Chapter 2), as far as is empirically certain, Laënnec was the first to use a stethoscope to systematically categorize the breath or lung, heart, and intestinal sounds he heard via mediate auscultation and to publish his findings for widespread dissemination and scrutiny. As Laënnec classified, "Various sounds, foreign to the natural respiratory murmur or resonance of the voice, may arise within the chest from various accidental causes: I shall class these under two heads—*the rattle* and *metallic tinkling.*"[20] What is rhetorically remarkable about Laënnec's classification work—however it was accepted [or not] by the medical community[21]—is that we can pinpoint when formalized medico-sonic knowledge began to enter modern medical and even public discourse: 1819 in France.

In the process, this medico-sonic knowledge demystified stethoscope-mediated auscultation and the body's sounds while simultaneously inviting physicians to participate in what can be described as an unintended, yet widespread, coordinated experiment and progymnasmatic event to test Laënnec's sonic findings. He presented those findings in *de l'auscultation médiate*, and when patrons and physicians bought the text, they could also purchase a stethoscope Laënnec made. Through this work, medical knowledge about the body's sounds—in this instance heart, intestine, or lung sounds—transforms the once rhetorically ineffable and coordinates it into more widely understood, permanent sonic understandings of the body primarily through two rhetorical devices: simile and metaphor. It is at this point where Laënnec harnesses distributed knowledge—like Edwin Hutchins's description of distributed cognition about Polynesian sailors navigating celestially via an astrolabe[22]—across civilizations and millennia—and provides widespread access to such sonic bodily understandings. It is transferred through the tandem experimentation provided to physicians with the *de l'auscultation médiate* (and its subsequent translations) text-stethoscope purchase. From here, sound in health and healing becomes more noticeable, engrained, and prominently integrated with technology. In this chapter, as well as the next, I use rhetoric to redescribe how healthcare technologies use sound in health, healing, and hospital contexts, including pedagogical ones.

When amplified, the body's sounds—the sounds of our lungs, hearts, and other organs—assist healthcare clinicians diagnose and provide care. Examined rhetorically, the care process reflects the paternalism that can exist between patients and their providers where physicians are privileged over patient autonomy and decision-making. The process draws from a similar rhetorical structure embedded in conventional healthcare systems—a source of real and rhetorical power privileging medically-sanctioned methods, such as medical devices, to *know about the body*, while disempowering the actual body, its functions, and its senses. I argue unintentional uses of healthcare technologies integrated with bodily sounds demonstrate most clearly sound's rhetorical power. In support of my position, I answer these questions:

- How does Laënnec use rhetoric in *de l'auscultation mediate* to create medico-sonic knowledge about the body? How does his use of rhetoric persist today?
- What modern health and healing technologies use sound diagnostically, prognostically, and therapeutically?
- How are unintentional uses of sound from healthcare technologies rhetorical?

Rhetoric, Sound, and Laënnec Then; Rhetoric and Sound Now

Although the content and comparisons of similes and metaphors through cultures and time vary, their rhetorical and pedagogical functions as medico-sonic learning tools persist. Rhetorically, Laënnec draws upon and unwittingly gathers sonic fragments from ancient health and healing systems and assembles them in his textual, sonic treatise, which can be understood with a stethoscope and familiarity with clinical knowledge and his cultural references and allusions. As his work garnered support and eventual widespread acceptance over the last two centuries, what resulted from Laënnec's work is a rhetorically powerful, influential entity capable of intentionally and unintentionally shaping bodies, their care, and actions. Laënnec gathered, harnessed, and coordinated medico-sonic knowledge for extended medical- or nursing-like progymnasmatic lessons achieved via using the stethoscope—a rhetorically powerful action that establishes an "audile technique"[23] as a physical assessment method in the Western biomedical health tradition. Through Laënnec, the body's sounds became rhetorically notable and widely knowable, all of which contributed to inscribing rhetorical power into sonic dimensions of Western biomedical understandings of health and healing, including even those that draw upon sound to diagnose and treat the body.

Using rhetoric and a stethoscope, Laënnec formalized sonic correlations between heart, intestine, and lung sounds with clinical conditions and diagnoses. His work provided a similar opportunity as Carl Linnaeus's binomial nomenclature or taxonomy of naming and classifying organisms by genus and species—organizing information for widespread dissemination, scientific discussion, and formal education. Linnaeus's work was also used as a tool to disseminate scientifically-supported ideas suggesting a hierarchy of humans that promoted anti-Black and ethnic racism, as well as colonization and justification for ethnic-based atrocities.[24] Laënnec's medico-sonic work did not provide a platform for weaponizing science against people and promoting White supremacy. Instead, Laënnec's work formalized knowledge and learning about sonic understandings of the body—medico-sonic knowledge later politically deployed in discourses about abortion and bodily autonomy.[25] Politically motivated, sonically amplified fetal heart sounds through ultrasound draw from a presumptive rhetorical power now inherent in Western biomedicine. A rhetorical power harnessed, then transformed from the ineffable to onomatopoeia and through simile and metaphor into Laënnec's standardized medico-sonic system to what it is today.

According to Jonathan Sterne, mediate auscultation was the first "audile technique"[26] or "set of culturally defined listening practices"[27] "where modern techniques of listening were developed and used."[28] However, without taking the ineffable sounds of the body and trying to put them into words through onomatopoeia, such as "debdeb," "rou" as roar, or "a mouth that roars," auscultation and percussion are without sound or voice, yet predate mediate auscultation as known audile techniques. Through Laënnec's creation of and work with the stethoscope, mediate auscultation would eventually develop into an indexed system of what Sterne dubbed "new medical semiotics."[29] Schafer would likely argue "new medical semiotics" rely upon sonological competence and training for proficient use—what I call the medico-sonic systematization of a rhetoric-sonic interplay or coaction. For example, Laënnec's work in *de l'auscultation médiate* painstakingly accounted for what the stethoscope heard and then interpreted as "diagnostic signs"[30]—the *crackling, crepitant, gurgling, sonorous, and whistling* of the lungs and other auscultatable organs. In the process, through medico-sonic knowledge the stethoscope provided, the sounds of bodies could be cataloged in a "sonic lexicon."[31] When Laënnec attempted to overcome ineffability—that is, the difficulty of putting these sounds into word—without onomatopoeia, he catalogued his quasi-objective diagnostic or clinical meaning using rhetoric's simile and standard metaphors. The reliance on simile and metaphor to describe the body's seemingly ineffable sounds rhetorically transforms the body's ineffable or onomatopoeiac sound from subjective and open to interpretation to standardized and sonically defined[32] (even with cultural, translational, and temporal interpretations). Laënnec provided an opportunity for other physicians to test his auditory observations by offering a stethoscope to purchase along with *de l'auscultation médiate*. By doing so, he directly contributed to harnessing and sharing medico-sonic knowledge about the body and the rhetorical, Western biomedical context for standardizing access and use of this kind of auditory-based sonic body knowledge.

User @BeautifulNursing—a registered nurse named Amanda—perhaps unwittingly builds upon Laënnec's medico-sonic knowledge and mediate auscultation integrated with social entertainment platform TikTok. According to Amanda, she is "Nurse w/a passion to help others" who makes "Nursing Cheat Sheets & Tools"[33]—pedagogical and clinical nursing tools for remembering or recalling information related to nursing education. Some of the cheat sheets and tools she makes are memory aids or mnemonics, such as intravenous therapy complications represented as PIE (Phlebitis, Infiltration, and Extravasation)[34] or medications needing verification by a second nurse as HICKOP [Heparin, Insulin, Chemotherapy, Potassium (periodic table abbreviation, K), Opioids, and Pediatric/neonate].[35,36]

In a 77 second video explaining lung sounds posted in 2021 viewed by more than 12 million and liked by over 2.2 million users, @BeautifulNursing draws upon audio and written descriptions of lung sounds as metaphors and similes with audio exemplifying those sounds. The video starts with a closeup of a stethoscope, which implies that metaphors and similes for the lung sounds presented in the video are heard through a stethoscope via mediate auscultation. For example, normal (vesicular) lung sounds sound like "AIR passing in and out"; coarse crackles—pneumonia, heart disease, cystic fibrosis, bronchitis—sounds like "shoveling large rocks" whereas fine crackles sound like the candy "pop rocks" or "slurping the last of your drink"; wheezing from allergies sounds like "blowing a musical horn"; pleural friction rub—inflammation of pleura—sounds like "walking on a creaky wooden floor"; rhonchi sounds like "snorkeling or snoring"; and stridor—croup—sounds like "a seal barking."[37]

Although I cannot account for the clinical accuracy of @BeautifulNursing's content, Laënnec's foundation of medico-sonic knowledge about the body's sounds that draw from culturally and temporally-dependent rhetorical devices are apparent. For example, Laënnec describes vesicular respiration sounds when

> applying the cylinder [stethoscope], with its funnel-shaped cavity open, to the breast of a healthy person, we hear, during inspiration and expiration, a slight but extremely distinct murmur, answering to the entrance of the air into, and its expulsion from, the air-cells of the lungs. This murmur may be compared to that produced by *a pair of bellows whose valve makes no noise, or, still better, to that emitted by a person in a deep and placid sleep, who makes now and then a profound inspiration.*[38]

Laënnec uses both rhetorical simile ("pair of bellows"—a device used to push out a strong current or blast of air) and metaphor ("emitted by a person in a deep and placid sleep … who makes now and then a profound inspiration"). When Laënnec published *de l'auscultation médiate* in 1819, it is likely most individuals reading Laënnec's work in either French or later English would be familiar with the role of a pair of bellows to provide a draught when starting or maintaining fire. Similarly, @BeautifulNursing draws upon allusion to popular culture in her simile description of fine crackles as "pop rocks" or "slurping the last of your drink." Conversely, Laënnec describes fine crackle or fine *râle*—a French word meaning rattle—or *rhoncus*—its Latin counterpart—as "the dry crepitous rhonchus, with large bubbles, or crackling"[39] that "entirely resembles the sound produced by blowing into a dried bladder."[40]

By "blowing into a dried bladder," it is likely Laënnec meant the bladder or organ of an animal or fish. When Laënnec described "the dry sibilous rhoncus" in *de l'auscultation médiate*, he wrote:

> sometimes it is like a prolonged whistle, flat or sharp, dull or loud; sometimes it's very momentary, and resembles the chirping of birds, the sound emitted by suddenly separating two portions of smooth oiled stone, or by the action of a small valve. The different kinds often exist together in different parts of the lungs, or successively in the same part. The peculiar nature of the sound, and the appearances on dissection seem to prove the sibilant rattle to be owing to minute portions of very vicid [sic] mucus obstructing, more or less completely, the small bronchial ramifications.[41]

In his description, Laënnec used simile ("like a prolonged whistle, flat or sharp, dull or loud") and metaphor ("chirping of birds, the sound emitted by suddenly separating two portions of smooth oiled stone, or by the action of a small valve"). Like @BeautifulNursing's simile comparing fine crackles to "pop rocks," Laënnec also relies on temporally- and culturally-situated shared knowledge to describe the body's lung sounds and what those lung sounds clinically and diagnostically indicate. In this case, Laënnec uses the rhetorical combination of simile and metaphor to sonically describe the "peculiar nature of the sound." I admit I am baffled by Laënnec's metaphor contained in "the sound emitted by suddenly separating two portions of smooth oiled stone"—I sonically imagine a wet suction-like sound. However, I am sonically familiar with @BeautifulNursing's rhetorical simile and allusion to fine crackles as "pop rocks" or "slurping the last of your drink [through a straw]"—I am quite confident I could hear and perhaps accurately identify fine crackles through mediate auscultation with rhetorical assistance from @BeautifulNursing's similes. Regardless of cultural knowledge or temporal orientation, Laënnec, @BeautifulNursing, and their metaphors and similes rely on rhetoric to interpret the sounds of the body and make them knowable to others for diagnosis, prediction, and treatment.

Diagnostic Uses of Sound

In addition to alerts and alarms and auscultation and percussion, sound provides many sources of medical data[42] through clinical physical examinations and diagnostic healthcare technologies. In many health systems, sound is used diagnostically to identify or confirm suspected ailments, conditions, and diseases. Although immediate or direct auscultation does not require a stethoscope, when used it allows for mediated auscultation and percussion. Yet, whether mediated with a stethoscope or not, through auscultation healthcare clinicians listen for heart, intestine, and lung sounds that possibly indicate health or disease within the body. In the process, auscultation or listening to the body assists healthcare clinicians in assessment and diagnosis. For example, by listening to the heart, an experienced clinician might hear a pericardial friction rub. As Leslie E. Tingle et al. explained, "The pericardial rub is best auscultated with the diaphragm of the stethoscope over the left lower sternal border in end expiration with the patient leaning forward. It has a rasping or creaking sound similar to leather rubbing against leather."[43] Tingle describes the rasping or creaking using a rhetorical device—metaphor—to describe a pericardial friction rub heart sound as similar to leather rubbing against leather.

In another example, pulmonary health might also be understood by mediating the triangle of lung auscultation. As Nazish Malik et al. described, the

> assessment of the thorax is a fundamental part of any physical examination as the location of many vital structures are in this region. On the dorsum of the thorax, there exists a relative thinning of the muscles that provide an essential anatomical landmark which aids clinicians during pulmonary auscultation and various thoracic procedures.[44]

Percussion is also assisted or unassisted by a stethoscope to assess the body. For example, abdominal percussion can be used during a physical examination. As Adrian Reuben described,

> expert percussion involves a series of sudden flicking strokes arising smoothly at the supple flexed wrist, so that the distal pad of the plexor hits the middle phalanx of the pleximeter smoothly and sharply, and withdraw immediately to prevent damping of the percussion notes. From their sound and tactile perception, the abdominal nodes can be categorized as resonant or tympanic due to air or gas; dull due to muscle, soft tissue, or an organ; or stony dull due to fluid. Malposition of the pleximeter and/or jerky, stiff, or irregular execution of the strike leads to erroneous findings on percussion.[45]

Lacking the clinical expertise of sonologically competent healthcare clinicians, the medico-sonic interpretations of the body these excerpts describe is clearly a valuable physical examination and assessment tool for understanding the health of bodies via auscultation and percussion. As diagnostic tools, using hearing ears—or sounds amplified via a digital stethoscope, such as medical student Alexandra Elaine who uses a wireless Bluetooth stethoscope that connects to her hearing aids for "super hearing"—to listen to the circulatory, digestive, and pulmonary systems provides easy-to-use physical assessment methods to assist clinicians as they assess and diagnose bodies. With the advent of the stethoscope and its broad, universal integration into conventional, science-based, allopathic Western health systems, the stethoscope in the ears of expert auscultating, percussing clinicians remains like Hutchins's astrolabe—a tool that provides access to accumulated knowledge and orients user cognition and sonic knowledge over time, especially when used alongside rhetorically-mediated medico-sonic knowledge of the body, such as examples from Laënnec and @BeautifulNursing.

Because of the growing knowledge of acoustical physics and other technological advances in healthcare, sound, its waves, and its affordances have been harnessed for its ability to use sound to see inside the body. In fact, the Acoustical Society of America's dedicated Biomedical Acoustics Technical Committee, formerly the Biomedical Ultrasound/Bioresponse to Vibration, is "concerned with the study of the interactions of acoustic waves with biological materials, including cells, tissues, organ systems and entire organisms."[46] Sometimes such "interactions of acoustic waves" with bodies is loud and noisy. Distinctive and unforgettable "loud knocking noises" for those who can hear,[i] MRI scanning offers an array of diagnostic capabilities.[47] An MRI relies on "strong magnetic fields and radio waves (radiofrequency energy) to make images. The signal in an MR image comes mainly from the protons in fat and water molecules in the body."[48] For example, "MRI gives health care providers useful information about a variety of conditions and diagnostic procedures including:

- abnormalities of the brain and spinal cord
- abnormalities in various parts of the body such as breast, prostate, and liver
- injuries or abnormalities of the joints
- the structure and function of the heart (cardiac imaging)
- areas of activation within the brain (functional MRI or fMRI)
- blood flow through blood vessels and arteries (angiography)
- the chemical composition of tissues (spectroscopy)

In addition to these diagnostic uses, MRI may also be used to guide certain interventional procedures."[49]

Ultrasound is a medical device like MRI, so it is under the regulatory jurisdiction of the Food and Drug Administration (FDA) in the United States. The FDA regulates and recommends uses of ultrasound imaging for healthcare clinicians, as well as approvals, suspensions, and revocations for medical devices and health technologies like ultrasound.[50] The FDA describes ultrasound as sonography that

uses high-frequency sound waves to view inside the body. Because ultrasound images are captured in real-time, they can also show movement of the body's internal organs as well as blood flowing through the blood vessels. Unlike X-ray imaging, there is no ionizing radiation exposure associated with ultrasound imaging.[51]

---

i After an MRI in May 2019, I described the sound of the MRI as wrenches and hammers cyclically spinning around in a tumbling clothes dryer.

Even in 2020, the FDA-approved novel uses of ultrasound imaging. For example, "the first cardiac ultrasound software that uses artificial intelligence (AI) to guide the user to capture quality diagnostic images" was approved for marketing.[52]

Without sound in health and healing, healthcare clinicians would be severely limited in their diagnostic capabilities (even with auscultation and percussion). The aforementioned diagnostic uses of sound in health and healing are not exhaustive and most do not require rhetoric-sonic interplay to function. However, auscultation and percussion, MRI, and ultrasound are widely known, used to diagnose, and indicate bodily status. Understandings from these diagnostic tools come from foundations in rhetorically enabled medico-sonic knowledge. These diagnostic uses of sound also demonstrate the various healthcare technologies and their power to know the body by looking into it with the help of sound, which results in synchresis—the confluence or merging of visual and audio.[53] The conflux or interplay of the sonic and the visual here are rhetorical. If feminist objectivity—as Donna J. Harraway points out—"allows us to become answerable for what we learn how to see,"[54] then what we can *see, rhetorically*—or better yet *sense*—is enabled and constructed by sound. Although helpful, the synchretic tools are operated by humans under what François Cooren theorized as *rhetorical ventriloquis*m—a kind of "vocal artifice."[55] Cooren defined it as "the various ways by which human interactants make certain entities (collectives, procedures, policies, ideologies, etc.) speak in their name and vice versa."[56] In the case of diagnostic technologies that rely on sound or synchresis, the MRI and ultrasound operate as powerful, directive vibrations within hospitals that provide insight into bodies. The insight depends on medico-sonic knowledge and semantic listening capabilities. Yet, such healthcare technologies possess the real and the rhetorical power to help, heal, and even harm.

Prognostic Uses of Sound

The diagnostic potential sound introduced through stethoscopes transformed from auscultation and percussion into more sophisticated diagnostic technologies like MRI and ultrasound imaging to prognostic technologies as well. Yet, before health technologies provided prognostic information based on sound, more common, less sophisticated methods—coughing and sneezing—also provided diagnostic information for physicians and prognostic information for individuals. Common respiratory symptoms related to infection, disease, and allergies often include cough, which clears out unwanted debris from lungs, and sneeze, which clears nasal passages. Anecdotally, years ago I saw a sign in a chiropractor's office during flu season that read "sneezing and coughing mean our bodies are working." When we sneeze or cough, we usually make a sound—the onomatopoeic "achoo" for a sneeze or "cough-cough" for, well, cough. Those sounds can indicate the health of the body or its work to make the body healthy by expelling some unwanted or unwelcome virus, bacteria, or debris. In another instance of cough as prognostic, individuals are sometimes asked by physicians to "turn and cough" to stimulate internal pressure and movement within the abdomen that allows physicians to check for inguinal hernia.

With the knowledge that sounds from sneezes and coughs can indicate health, infection, and disease, sonic healthcare technologies mimic the sonic qualities of our bodies to predict or provide prognostic information. For example, researchers used audio-detected cough frequency via CoughSense software as one of several measures to estimate tuberculosis transmission risk.[57] Created at the University of Washington in Shwetak Patel's Ubiquitous Computer (UbiComp) lab that "develops innovative sensing systems for real world applications in health, sustainability, and novel interactions," CoughSense preserves an individual's privacy while using strategically placed microphones to detect and record personal or networked cough frequency for later analysis via AI.[58] Researchers estimated Mycobacterium tuberculosis (Mtb) transmission by measuring patient and environmental data, collecting patient movements, cough frequency, and clinical data, and measuring indoor carbon dioxide (CO_2) levels, relative humidity, and Mtb genomes in the air. In combination, cough frequency—a sound-related respiratory symptom of tuberculosis infection—and measuring Mtb genomes in the air (spread by cough) were used to estimate or predict Mtb transmission.

Regarding senses and sound, UbiComp is a unique lab. UbiComp "focuses on leveraging the ubiquity" of "commodity sensors, such as cameras or microphones on smartphones, wearables, or with purpose-specific sensors given added signal processing" to detect biosignals associated with certain conditions, "such as anemia, jaundice, tuberculosis, influenza, and traumatic brain injuries."[59] Among others, UbiComp also develops sensors, such as SpiroCall or SpiroSmart, that use mobile phone microphones to remotely estimate lung function using sound[60] and LuckyChirp uses cascaded sonar modeling to remotely estimate respiration with Google Nest Hub and Pixel 4 (or like devices).[61] With remote sound detection and local replication, the UbiComp lab also relies on medico-sonic understandings of the body and common commodities, such as smartphones, to harness and replicate sounds our bodies naturally produce to predict what those sounds might mean when integrating the sonic with healthcare technologies and mobile health apps. Prognostic uses of sound in health and healing contexts tether to common technologies, such as smartphones. The UbiComp lab appears devoted to using everyday items for sensing our bodies and making conventional, science-based allopathic Western biomedical care decisions about what those everyday items sense.

Therapeutic Uses of Sound

Sound is used to understand and diagnose the body and make predictions about what the body's sounds indicate; sound is also used to treat the body. In Western biomedicine, in addition to their diagnostic capabilities, ultrasound and MRI are dually known for their therapeutic capabilities as well. Certain CAM health systems also rely on sound and vibration as therapies to treat and heal bodies. For example, the Japanese practice of forest bathing (Japanese: *shinrin-yoku*) relies upon the sounds of nature to promote health and happiness.[62] As another example, tuning forks are used as a component of music therapy.

The now defunct (2013–2018) open-access *Journal of Therapeutic Ultrasound* was established "to accelerate the development of focused ultrasound and its adoption in the clinic" through "reaching audiences around the world … [and] play[ing] a key role in advancing clinical applications of therapeutic ultrasound."[63] Therapeutic uses of ultrasound applications at low powers have been used widely since the 1950s in physio or physical therapy contexts to treat conditions such as tendinitis and bursitis.[64] The FDA-approved uses for ultrasound therapy range from warming tissues with portable handheld applicators to regional heating with multielement applicators as cancer therapy.[65] Other uses of ultrasound therapy include glaucoma relief, laparoscopic tissue ablation, skin tissue tightening, plantar fasciitis, lens removal, adipose tissue removal, transdermal drug delivery, and bone fracture healing.[66]

When used therapeutically, ultrasound deposits energy "in tissue to induce various biological effects."[67] Since there are broad and evolving therapeutic uses for ultrasound and no ionizing or harmful radiation from it, ultrasound devices are found in an array healthcare practitioner offices if financially feasible, such as physician or chiropractor offices. Ultrasound imaging is a versatile therapeutic tool for healthcare clinicians to "evaluate, diagnose, and treat medical conditions" through various healthcare technologies, such as

- abdominal ultrasound (to visualize abdominal tissues and organs),
- bone sonometry (to assess bone fragility),
- breast ultrasound (to visualize breast tissue),
- Doppler fetal heart rate monitors (to listen to the fetal heartbeat),
- Doppler ultrasound (to visualize blood flow through a blood vessel, organs, or other structures),
- echocardiogram (to view the heart),
- fetal ultrasound (to view the fetus in pregnancy),
- ultrasound-guided biopsies (to collect a sample of tissue),
- ophthalmic ultrasound (to visualize ocular structures), and
- ultrasound-guided needle placement (in blood vessels or other tissues of interest).[68]

As another example, in 2020 the FDA also approved a "high intensity focused ultrasound (HIFU), magnetic-resonance [MR] guided, ablation system for the treatment of osteoid osteomas, a type of tumor, in the extremities."[69] Guided by MRI and treated by ultrasound, a clinical trial "Therapeutic Magnetic Resonance Imaging (MRI)-Guided High Intensity Focused Ultrasound (HIFU) Ablation of Uterine Fibroids" was registered in 2009 with the FDA to use MRI and HIFU as a therapeutic treatment.[70] Eventually the MRI-HIFU method was shown to effectively treat "uterine fibroids, palliation of bone pain, ablation of the prostate and treatment of essential tremor."[71]

Beyond Western biomedicine, there are less technologically-invasive therapeutic uses of sound in health and healing. For instance, take *shinrin-yoku*—forest bathing—or its offspring, forest therapy. Both rely upon the sounds of nature to promote health and happiness and encourage individuals to bathe in the natural sounds of the forest. Forest therapy has been described as "unlike a hike or guided nature walk aimed at identifying trees or birds, forest therapy relies on trained guides, who set a deliberately slow pace and invite people to experience the pleasures of nature through all of their senses," including sound.[72] Or, take the YouTube-originating Autonomous Sensory Meridian Response (ASMR) that has been described as a "brain-gasm" stimulated by comforting visuals and sounds, such as the sound of brushing long, dry hair with a hard-handled plastic-bristle brush or listening to women whisper.[73] In "How A.S.M.R. Became a Sensation," Jamie Lauren Keiles explains to her *New York Times* readers that she "spent at least 200 hours on the [ASMR YouTube] site, watching women chew gum, swallow octopus sashimi, simulate eye exams, turn pages of books and peel dried glue off artificial ears ... [She] watched a two-hour recording of hair-dryer sounds."[74] Although Keiles indicates that she watched and listened to the videos, a draw for ASMR is their sonic qualities and the relaxing tingles ASMR viewers report as a result from watching or listening. ASMR is a relatively new sonic therapy; however, in the short time that it is been used (since 2009), ASMR has "begun to find broader appeal as a sleep aid, an alternative to guided meditation and a drug-free, online version of Xanax."[75]

Music as therapy or music therapy uses sound and music to heal, and its roots go back at least as far as ancient Greece. In *Sound and the Ancient Senses*—the final addition to a series on the senses in antiquity—Colin Webster's chapter-length contribution to the volume, "The Soundscape of Ancient Greek Healing," noted that Hippocratic medical practices often approached sound as "treating the body as an echoing chamber of noises to be heard, discerned and understood."[76] Webster also noted that "from our earliest evidence, music was part of medicine."[77] Ancient Greeks Aesclepius and Hippocrates used music to treat mental and physical ailments,[78] yet music was "cleaved from the physician's toolkit" by the close of the fifth century BCE.[79] Some modern examples of music therapy are listening to or playing an instrument with a music therapist. Adrienne Santos-Longhurst described music therapy that

uses calibrated metal tuning forks to apply specific vibrations to different parts of the body. This can help release tension and energy, and promote emotional balance. It supposedly works similarly to acupuncture, using sound frequencies for point stimulation instead of needles.[80]

Santos-Longhurst also names other kinds of music therapy, such as guided meditation, neurologic music therapy (e.g., prior to surgery to manage anxiety), the Bonny Method of Guided Imagery and Music that uses classical music to manage stress, the Nordoff–Robbins sound healing method administered by musicians to treat children experiencing developmental delays, for example, and binaural beats or brainwave entrainment. As an example of the latter, the United Kingdom-based Marconi Union track "Weightless"[ii] is touted as the most relaxing song in the world.

There are other forms of sound therapy that involve ancient musical instruments: Tibetan singing bowls and digeridoos. In an observational study from the *Journal of Evidence-based Complementary & Alternative Medicine*, Tibetan singing bowl meditations reduced tension, anger, fatigue, and depressed mood among participants.[81] Tibetan singing bowls are made "of a combination of metal alloys ... originally used by Tibetan monks for spiritual ceremonies."[82] In a study comparing silent meditation with didgeridoo meditation, participants reported experiencing more relaxation than their silent meditation counterparts.[83] A didgeridoo (Aborigine: yiḍaki) is a musical instrument used for at least the last 1,500 years by Aboriginal people in now northern Australia; the instrument relies on circular breathing and vibration to produce sound.[84] Although Tibetan or Himalayan singing bowls and didgeridoo or yiḍaki are not commonly used in conventional, science-based allopathic Western biomedical healthcare as a treatment for conditions or diseases and the studies referenced here are just two, the sounds produced by these ancient instruments show promise as recognized sonic therapeutic methods for intentionally reducing stress and promoting health and healing.

Harnessing Rhetoric's Power by Unintentional Uses of Sonic Healthcare Technologies

The aforementioned sonic diagnostic, prognostic, and therapeutic methods intentionally use sound to assist healthcare clinicians to understand or assess the health of bodies (e.g., stethoscope, ultrasound), provide prognostic information (e.g., tuberculosis transmission risk), and treatments and therapies (e.g., MRI-guided ultrasound, tuning forks, forest therapy). However, there are other intentional sources of sound, especially in conventional, science-based

ii Although anecdotal, throughout my work for this book, I listened to Marconi Union's "Weightless" and "Akihabara (Electric Town)" on multiple productive occasions before and during writing, and the music did indeed provide unexpected relaxation and general feelings of well-being.

allopathic Western biomedical healthcare spaces, such as hospitals and the NICU at the center of the next chapter, when the sounds of the body are amplified via healthcare technologies; unintentional noises made by these technologies influence actions and discipline bodies, such as responding to a physiological monitor's false alarm, in those and other healthcare contexts.

Unintentional means the by-product or purpose of using the healthcare technology is not diagnostic, prognostic, or therapeutic—the use is not primarily or wholly medical. The rhetorical power derived in contexts when sound is used unintentionally emanates from a dual strength originating when the body's sounds integrate with medical devices within conventional, science-based, allopathic Western medical contexts. Whether the body's sounds rhetorically work to assist healthcare clinicians care for patients or not, the paternalism that exists between patients and their providers draws from a similar rhetorical structure embedded in conventional healthcare systems. The location when such rhetorical power is wielded positions one agent superior, one inferior. In paternalistic medical contexts, the physician is the former, the patient the latter. When tracked onto conventional, science-based allopathic Western medicine, such paternalistic rhetorical structures position knowing about the body above the body and its senses. Where the sonic is concerned, the hospital and its medically-sanctioned methods to know about the body— healthcare technologies and medical devices—yield rhetorical power over the bodies they rely on to make sounds from and the sounds they amplify.

To be certain, sound from healthcare technologies enable care and allow for life, health, and healing; however, the following rhetorical examination of the unintentional by-products and surprising uses of sound are meant to provide a deeper, more nuanced understanding of its rhetorical work and power. In some cases, such as alarm fatigue, the body's sounds are amplified through healthcare technologies and allowed to sonically disperse in health and healing contexts mostly unchecked and sometimes causing great harm. As another example, ultrasound functions as a diagnostic and therapeutic healthcare technology for the management of kidney stones. Sound is used by ultrasound to interact with biological materials to mold health and healing. However, MRI can simultaneously contribute to efforts toward health and healing, and auditorily stun the individual who experiences it, "worsening anxiety, [and] triggering claustrophobia."[85] Of course, anxiety and claustrophobia are not diagnostic, prognostic, or therapeutic uses of the MRI or its use of sound; these are an MRI's sonic, unintentional, unwelcome by-products.

In Shaheen E. Lakhan's case report, Lakhan described a person who experienced post-traumatic stress disorder (PTSD) from receiving an MRI. Lakhan noted that

the patient experienced acute agitation, fear, anxiety, tachypnea, tachycardia with palpitations, and dizziness. He felt intense surface heat over segments of his body and very loud noises. He perceived impending serious bodily harm by the scanner. The scan was aborted at the lumbar spine, and cervical and thoracic spine was unremarkable. The patient's pain resolved in the weeks following with over the counter analgesics, however, he developed increased arousal, re-experiencing the event, persistent avoidance, and significant psychosocial impairment.[86]

According to Lakhan, "This is the first published report of PTSD following 'traumatic' MRI."[87] There are other reported unintentional effects from MRI. For example, take Sedat Alibek et al.'s "Acoustic Noise Reduction in MRI Using Silent Scan: An Initial Experience." In their technical note, Alibek et al. pointed out that MRI noise "is one of the main sources of patient complaints and discomfort."[88] Furthermore, in their review article, "Auditory Noise Associated with MR Procedures," authors reported noise from MRIs contribute to an array of issues for people, ranging from "simple annoyance" to "difficulties in verbal communication, heightened anxiety, temporary hearing loss, and potential permanent hearing impairment."[89] Sonic MRI by-products are unintentional, yet likely predictable.

In the United States, the quintessential, conventional, science-based, allopathic Western medical context—the hospital—is a noisy space where ubiquitous healthcare technologies, such as physiological monitors and ventilators, surveil a body's vital signs—pulse, body temperature, and breathing rate. In the process, these healthcare technologies make sounds that contribute to ambient (i.e., environmental[90]) noise that impacts patient care. In some cases, healthcare technology sounds resulted in alarm fatigue.[91] Alarm fatigue happens when nurses are "exposed to an excessive number of alarms, which can result in desensitization to alarms and missed alarms."[92] Alarm fatigue has been associated with negatively impacting patient care[93] and causing patient deaths.[94] In fact, between 2005 and 2008, the FDA reported that alarm fatigue caused "566 alarm-related deaths"[95]; and 73 others died due to alarm desensitization (i.e., alarm fatigue) between March and June 2010[96–97] from medical devices or technologies.

Due to the heavy reliance on Western biomedicine for care during the COVID-19 pandemic, healthcare clinicians and their expertise have been called upon in unprecedented ways. Part of their work—as user @Nurse_Sushi previously demonstrated in Chapter 1—involves responding to purposeful auditory alarms (and listening to the alarms when there's nothing to be done) linked to a person's physiological process sonically amplified through a monitor or other healthcare technology. In "Alarm fatigue and moral distress in ICU nurses in COVID-19 pandemic," authors concluded nurses in Iran should have practical training courses on alarm management to reduce alarm fatigue.[98]

MRI noise and alarm fatigue as by-products are unintentional. However, when the purpose of using the healthcare technology or medical device is not diagnostic, prognostic, or therapeutic, it is medically unintentional or without medical intent. In the United States, an example of a medically unintentional use of sound occurs when ultrasound is used to deter and prohibit abortions and discipline the bodies of people who seek abortions. There are two distinct ways that ultrasound is used to influence and discipline bodies who seek abortions. First, prior to an abortion, an ultrasound technician can be required to sonically amplify fetal heart[99] sounds. In certain states, such as Kentucky prior to the Supreme Court of the United States overturning Roe vs. Wade, physicians were required to describe fetal ultrasound images while sonically amplifying fetal heart sounds.[100] The Kentucky abortion law "require[d] doctors to give a detailed description of fetal ultrasound images, including 'the presence of external members and internal organs.' Doctors are also required to make the fetal heartbeat audible if they can."[101] The second distinct way the anti-abortion movement co-opted ultrasound to deter abortion and discipline bodies is through a genre of specific abortion-prohibiting state laws identified as "heartbeat bills." Heartbeat bills indicate that once a fetus or embryo heartbeat can be sonically amplified via ultrasound, a person cannot legally receive an abortion. In the United States since 2011, state-level antiabortion legislation denying abortions to pregnant people has appeared throughout the country.[102] Without the sonic amplification of fetal heart sounds, this unintentional use of ultrasound and its sonic capabilities would not be possible.

Amanda Nell Edgar offers one example of the confluence of rhetoric, material variables, sound, the body, and the unintentional, non-medical use of healthcare technology. Edgar notes the sonogram was developed from SONAR—a sonic naval technology.[103] Sonography's deployment in abortion and fetal personhood contexts uses the visual and the sonic—or synchresis—to produce an "image based on the return of … sound waves through the [fetal] body, providing a technologically advanced means of listening to interior organs, a technique known as auscultation" and

> while … Doppler technology … allows doctors to auscultate fetal heartbeats [it] is not inherently related to the sonogram, they are very often discussed in tandem and linked together in discussion of prenatal examinations and … mandatory examinations preceding abortions in many states.[104]

Edgar's analysis of the "Heartbeat Bill" in Ohio provides an example of the rhetorical power of sound in abortion contexts to act as a powerful influence. The Heartbeat Bill also aims to harness ultrasound's sonic power and discipline bodies. Fetal auscultation—the fetal heartbeat—overpowers pregnant people's voices by amplifying a sonogram's sound, a healthcare technology that relies on sound's material role in our health and healing, yet in these contexts is powerfully deployed to discipline.

In an analysis of Georgia state antiabortion legislation on the fetal heartbeat, "a narrative analysis of antiabortion testimony and legislative debate related to Georgia's fetal 'heartbeat' abortion ban," found that "the use of the 'heartbeat' [was] an indicator of life and therefore personhood."[105] It seems a logical analytical finding from the unintentional—or not diagnostic, prognostic, or therapeutic—use of ultrasound. Clearly, ultrasound is purposefully and powerfully used; however, from a medical standpoint, the use of ultrasound is co-opted and used for a purpose beyond a conventional, science-based, allopathic Western medical one. In a way, it is a rhetorical call back to ancient Egyptian onomatopoeia and "debdeb"—the sound of the fetal heart as an indicator of life and health. The use of fetal heart sounds and their amplification takes the ineffable and deploys the sonic amplification rhetorically and politically to shape actions and emotions and discipline bodies. In the process, the heart sounds become persuasive in abortion contexts, strengthening or weakening resolve or even used as the method to deter or criminalize. Whatever the outcome, the effective use of ultrasound's sonic dimensions draws upon ultrasound's rhetorical power and power to discipline bodies, which emanates from its intended (and FDA-sanctioned) diagnostic and therapeutic uses.

Sound and a Neonatal Health Technology

Since the next chapter examines sound and its functions in a NICU, sound used as an alarm for a NICU technology over one hundred years ago is significant. In the first neonatology textbook *Premature and Congenitally Diseased Infants,* Chicago physician Julius Hess narrated the history of incubators. He indicated that

> [Charles Edward] Hearson introduced automatic temperature regulation within the incubator. His apparatus was so constructed as to set off *an electric alarm clock* [Figure 3.2] when the maximum temperature desired was past. This apparatus was modified by Eustache who attempted to attach automatic gas or oil-heating apparatus to the so-called "thermostat nurse of Hearson."[106] (emphasis added)

"An electric alarm clock" alerting clinicians about a patient's physiological status is unremarkable, given their proliferation in conventional, science-based, allopathic Western health contexts, such as hospital rooms, today. What is worthy of note involves introducing sound as an alarm in a NICU context. Furthermore, sonically alerting clinicians seems at-odds with predominant thinking that infants need to sleep. If sleep is best (for most) under quiet conditions, sound as an alarm is baffling and demonstrates priority for medical or clinical attention and action. Thus, as Chapter 4 scrutinizes, the introduction of audible alarm sounds and noises in a well-known sleeping context—a space occupied by snoozing infants—appears to be at cross-purposes.

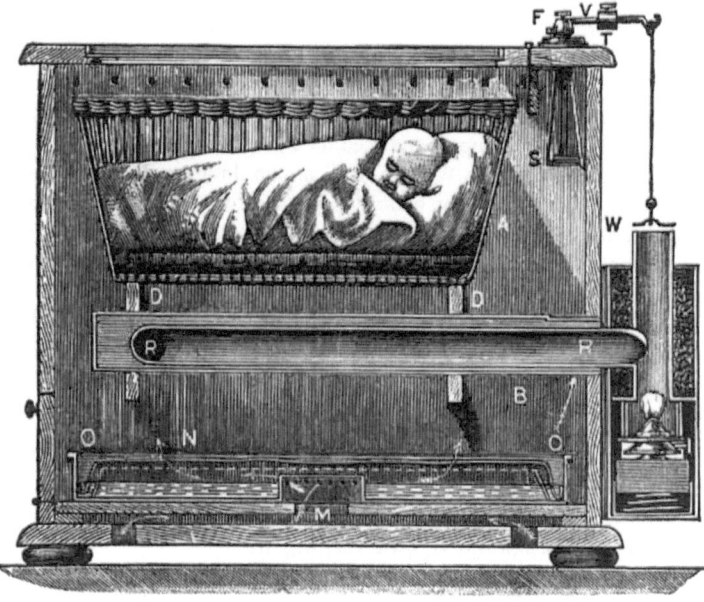

Figure 3.2 Hearson's thermostatic nurse incubator.[107] The letters indicate noteworthy functions Hearson developed unrelated to its appearance here.

Notes

1 Debra Hawhee and Christa J. Olson. "Pan-historiography: The Challenges of Writing History across Time and Space," in *Theorizing Histories of Rhetoric*, ed. Michelle Ballif (Carbondale, IL: Southern Illinois University Press, 2013), 90–105.
2 Rachel Hajar, "The Art of Listening," *Heart Views* 13, no. 1 (January–March 2012): 24, https://doi.org/10.4103/1995-705X.96668.
3 Noreen Iftikhar, "What is Allopathic Medicine?," *Healthline*, last reviewed on May 28, 2019, https://www.healthline.com/health/allopathic-medicine.
4 Rachel Hajar, "The Art of Listening," 24.
5 Hawhee and Olson, "Pan-historiography," 90.
6 Charles Bazerman, *The Languages of Edison's Light* (Cambridge, MA: MIT Press, 1999), 335.
7 Hutchins, *Cognition in the Wild*, 1995.
8 International Museum of Surgical Science (@surgicalmuseum), "Before the stethoscope, doctors had to press their ears directly against a patient's chest to hear their lungs! In 1816, French doctor René Laënnec felt uncomfortable with the practice and invented the first stethoscope, a long wooden tube that amplified sound," Twitter, April 29, 2020, 4:53 p.m., https://twitter.com/surgicalmuseum/status/1255616307082510342?lang=en.
9 Wikimedia, 2008, "Stethoscopes," Wikimedia Foundation. Last modified August 11, 2008. https://commons.wikimedia.org/wiki/User: Stethoscopes.

10 Forbes, "A Treatise on the Diseases," 4–5. Emphasis added.

11 Jenny Edbauer, "Unframing Models of Public Distribution: From Rhetorical Situation to Rhetorical Ecologies," *Rhetoric Society Quarterly* 35, no. 4 (Fall 2005): 7.

12 Ibid., 17.

13 Alaimo, Stacy, Susan Henkman, and Susan J. Hekman, eds. *Material Feminisms* (Bloomington, IN: Indiana University Press, 2008).

14 Ibid., 3.

15 Forbes, "A Treatise on the Diseases," 6.

16 Ibid., 537.

17 Alexandra Elaine. @alexandraelaineadams. "Disability is a superpower #foryou #foryourpage #fyp #medicine #medicalschool #medicalstudent #doctor #nhs #uk #deaf #blind #deafblind #disability #disabilitytiktok #disabilityawareness #education #advocate #misconception #mythbusters #anythingispossible #believeinyourself #superpower #superhero #achieveyourdreams #achieveyourgoals #lifegoals #rolemodel #humanity" TikTok. May 24, 2022. https://vm.tiktok.com/ZMNjpqQke/?k=1

18 Alexandra Elaine. @alexandraelaineadams. "Misconceptions on being a deafblind medical student #foryou #foryourpage #fyp #medicine #medicalstudent #doctor #nhs #healthcare #deafblind #deaf #blind #disability #disabilityawareness #education #advocate #misconception #breakingbarriers #mythbusters." TikTok. May 11, 2022. https://vm.tiktok.com/ZMNjsMYPh/?k=1

19 Thinklabs One, "Audio Power," para. 1, https://www.thinklabs.com/audio-power

20 Forbes, "A Treatise on the Diseases," 49.

21 Jacalyn M. Duffin, "The Medical Philosophy of R.T.H. Laënnec (1781–1826)," *History and Philosophy of the Life Sciences* 8, no. 2 (1986): 197. http://www.jstor.org/stable/23328661.

22 Edwin Hutchins. *Cognition in the Wild* (Cambridge, MA: MIT Press, 1995).

23 Jonathan Sterne, *The Audible Past* (Durham, NC: Duke University Press, 2003), https://doi.org/10.1515/9780822384250-toc.

24 Ibram X. Kendi, *Stamped from the Beginning: The Definitive History of Racist Ideas in America* (New York: Nation Books, 2016).

25 Amanda Nell Edgar, "The Rhetoric of Auscultation: Corporeal Sounds, Mediated Bodies, and Abortion Rights," *Quarterly Journal of Speech* 103, no. 4 (2017): 350–71.

26 Jonathan Sterne, *The Audible Past*.

27 Justin Eckstein, "Easy Listening: Spreading and the Role of the Ear in Debating," *Sounding Out* (blog), September 17, 2012, para. 5, https://soundstudiesblog.com/2012/09/17/easy-listening-spreading-and-the-role-of-the-ear-in-debating.

28 Sterne, *The Audible Past*, 137.

29 Ibid., 128.

30 Ibid., 129.

31 Ibid., 128.

32 Hippocrates: "He also described a sound in the chest which he compared to 'a creak like that of leather' probably pleural or pericardial friction" (James Alexander Lindsay, "Some Hints from the Old Physicians: An Address Delivered before the Bradford Medico-Chirurgical Society, October 17th, 1923," *British Medical Journal* 2, no. 3284 (December 1923): 1078.

33 @BeautifulNursing. 2022. "Nurse w/ a passion to help others Nursing Cheat Sheets & Tool." TikTok, July 21, 2022. https://www.tiktok.com/@beautifulnursing.

34 @BeautifulNursing. 2022. "IV Therapy Complications #fyp #foryou #nurse #nclex #FilmTeyvatIslands #ShowUrGrillSkillz. TikTok, July 19, 2022. https://www.tiktok.com/@beautifulnursing/video/7121832184586997034

35 @BeautifulNursing. 2022. "NCLEX TIP: HIGH ALERT MEDS #fyp #foryou #nurse #nursingstudent #nursingschool #nclex #nclextips #MadewithKAContest #PerfectPrideMovement #xyzbca #medtok #medmonday #nclexprep #nursinghacks #nclexhacks."TikTok, June 7, 2022. https://www.tiktok.com/@beautifulnursing/video/7106281561514954030

36 As several commenters point out—and as I show in the next chapter—high alert medications can differ state by state and hospital ward by hospital ward. For this reason, the items listed in this mnemonic are likely only accurate in specific and not all contexts.

37 @BeautifulNursing. 2022. "LUNG SOUNDS #fyp #foryou #nurse #nursingschool #medical." TikTok. June 24, 2021. https://www.tiktok.com/@beautifulnursing/video/6977189254690589958

38 Forbes, "A Treatise on the Diseases," 34. Emphasis added.

39 Ibid., 55.

40 Ibid., 56.

41 Ibid., 61.

42 Mattern, "Urban Auscultation," para. 10.

43 Leslie E. Tingle, Daniel Molina, and Charles Calvert, "Acute Pericarditis," *American Family Physician* 76, no. 10 (2007): 1511.

44 Nazish Malik, Brandon Tedder, and Michael R. Zemaitis, *Anatomy, Thorax, Triangle of Auscultation* (Treasure Island, FL: StatPearls Publishing, 2021), para. 1, https://pubmed.ncbi.nlm.nih.gov/30969656.

45 Adrian Reuben, "Examination of the Abdomen," *Clinical Liver Disease* 7, no. 6 (June 2016), 147, https://aasldpubs.onlinelibrary.wiley.com/doi/pdf/10.1002/cld.556.

46 Acoustical Society of America, "About the BATC," para. 2, https://tcbaasa.org.

47 U.S. Food and Drug Administration, "MRI: Benefits and Risks," current as of December 9, 2017, para. 4, https://www.fda.gov/radiation-emitting-products/mri-magnetic-resonance-imaging/benefits-and-risks.

48 U.S. Food and Drug Administration, "MRI (Magnetic Resonance Imaging)," current as of August 29, 2018, para. 1, https://www.fda.gov/radiation-emitting-products/medical-imaging/mri-magnetic-resonance-imaging.

49 U.S. Food and Drug Administration, "MRI," para. 1–2.

50 U.S. Food and Drug Administration, "Ultrasound Imaging," current as of September 28, 2020, https://www.fda.gov/radiation-emitting-products/medical-imaging/ultrasound-imaging.

51 Ibid., para. 1–2.

52 U.S. Food and Drug Administration, "FDA News Release: FDA Authorizes Marketing of First Cardiac Ultrasound Software that Uses Artificial Intelligence to Guide User," February 7, 2020, para. 1, https://www.fda.gov/news-events/press-announcements/fda-authorizes-marketing-first-cardiac-ultrasound-software-uses-artificial-intelligence-guide-user.

53 Michel Chion, "The Three Listening Modes." Jonathan Sterne, ed. *The Sound Studies Reader* (New York: Routledge, 2012), 48–53.

54 Donna Harraway, "Situated Knowledges: The Science Question in Feminism and the Privilege of Partial Perspective," *Feminist Studies* 14, no. 3 (2013): 583.

55 Jonathan Sterne, *The Audible Past* (Durham, NC: Duke University Press, 2003), 492, https://doi.org/10.1515/9780822384250-toc.

56 Cooren, "The Selection of Agency," 23–24.

57 Kathrin Zürcher, Julien Riou, Carl Morrow, Marie Ballif, Anastasia Koch, Simon Bertschinger, Digby F. Warner et al., "Estimating Tuberculosis Transmission Risks in a Primary Care Clinic in South Africa: Modeling of Environmental and Clinical Data," *The Journal of Infectious Diseases* 225, no. 9 (2022): 1642–52.

58 UbiCompLab, "The Ubiquitous Computing Lab develops innovative sensing systems for real world applications in health, sustainability, and novel interactions," https://ubicomplab.cs.washington.edu/

59 UbiCompLab, "About the Lab," 2. https://ubicomplab.cs.washington.edu/pdfs/lab/ubicomplab-flyer.pdf

60 UbiCompLab, "SpiroCall: Measuring Lung Function over a Phone Call," https://ubicomplab.cs.washington.edu/publications/spirocall/

61 UbiCompLab, "LuckyChirp: Opportunistic Respiration Sensing Using Cascaded Sonar on a Commodity Device," https://ubicomplab.cs.washington.edu/publications/luckychirp/

62 Karin Evans, "Why Forest Bathing Is Good for Your Health," *Greater Good Magazine*, August 20, 2018, para. 6, https://greatergood.berkeley.edu/article/item/why_forest_bathing_is_good_for_your_health.

63 Robert Muratore and Arik Hananel, "The *Journal of Therapeutic Ultrasound*: Broadening Knowledge in a Rapidly Growing Field," *Journal of Therapeutic Ultrasound* 1, no. 1 (2013): 1–2, https://jtultrasound.biomedcentral.com/track/pdf/10.1186/2050-5736-1-1.pdf.

64 Douglas L. Miller, Nadine B. Smith, Michael R. Bailey, Gregory J. Czarnota, Kullervo Hynynen, Inder Raj S. Makin, and Bioeffects Committee of the American Institute of Ultrasound in Medicine, "Overview of Therapeutic Ultrasound Applications and Safety Considerations," *Journal of Ultrasound in Medicine* 31, no. 4 (2012): 623.

65 Ibid., 624.

66 Ibid., 624. These authors provide an overview of the broad uses of therapeutic ultrasound in their article, 626–628.

67 Ibid., 623.

68 U.S. Food and Drug Administration, "Ultrasound Imaging."

69 U.S. Food and Drug Administration, "Summary of Safety and Probable Benefit," HDEH190003, https://www.accessdata.fda.gov/cdrh_docs/pdf19/H190003B.pdf.

70 U.S. National Library of Medicine, "Therapeutic Magnetic Resonance Imaging (MRI)-Guided High Intensity Focused Ultrasound (HIFU) Ablation of Uterine Fibroids," ClinicalTrials.gov, April–December 2009, https://clinicaltrials.gov/ct2/show/NCT00897897.

71 Florian Siedek, Sin Yuin Yeo, Edwin Heijman, Olga Grinstein, Grischa Bratke, Carola Heneweer, Michael Puesken, Thorsten. Persigehl, David Maintz, and Holger Grüll, "Magnetic Resonance-Guided High-Intensity Focused Ultrasound (MR-HIFU): Technical Background and Overview of Current Clinical Applications (Part 1), *Rofo* 191, no. 6 (June 2019), para. 3, https://doi.org/10.1055/a-0817-5645.

72 Susan Abookire, "Can Forest Therapy Enhance Health and Well-Being?," *Harvard Health Blog*, May 29, 2020, para. 2, https://www.health.harvard.edu/blog/can-forest-therapy-enhance-health-and-well-being-2020052919948.

73 Jamie Lauren Keiles, "How A.S.M.R. Became a Sensation," *New York Times Magazine*, April 4, 2019, para. 4, https://www.nytimes.com/2019/04/04/magazine/how-asmr-videos-became-a-sensation-youtube.html.

74 Ibid., para. 14.

75 Ibid., para. 25.

76 Webster, Colin. "The Soundscape of Ancient Greek Healing," in *Sound and the Ancient Senses* (Routledge, 2018), 109–29.

77 Ibid., 110.

78 Christos Kleisiaris, Chrisanthos Sfakianakis, and Ioanna Papathanasiou, "Health Care Practices in Ancient Greece: The Hippocratic Ideal," *Journal of Medical Ethics and History of Medicine* 7, no. 6 (2014), para. 9, https://www.ncbi.nlm.nih.gov/pmc/articles/PMC4263393.

79 Webster, "The Soundscape of Ancient Greek Healing," 110.
80 Adrienne Santos-Longhurst, "The Uses and Benefits of Music Therapy," *Healthline*, January 27, 2020, para. 14, https://www.healthline.com/health/sound-healing.
81 Tamara L. Goldsby, Michael E. Goldsby, Mary McWalters, and Paul J. Mills, "Effects of Singing Bowl Sound Meditation on Mood, Tension, and Well-Being: An Observational Study," *Journal of Evidence-Based Complementary & Alternative Medicine* 22, no. 3 (2017): 401–6.
82 Ibid., 401.
83 Kamaira Hartley Phillips, Carrie E. Brintz, Kevin Moss, and Susan A. Gaylord, "Didgeridoo Sound Meditation for Stress Reduction and Mood Enhancement in Undergraduates: A Randomized Controlled Trial," *Global Advances in Health and Medicine* 8 (2019): 2164956119879367.
84 Gauthier Aubé. "The Origins of the Didgeridoo: The Aborigines of Australia," Wakademy, January 25, 2021. https://www.wakademy.online/en/blog/aboriginal-culture/the-origins-of-the-didgeridoo-the-aborigines-of-australia/.
85 Shaheen Lakahn, "3T MRI Induced Post-Traumatic Stress Disorder: A Case Report," *International Archives of Medicine* 5, no. 27 (2012): 1, https://www.ncbi.nlm.nih.gov/pmc/articles/PMC3496599/pdf/1755-7682-5-27.pdf.
86 Ibid., 1.
87 Ibid., 2.
88 Sedat Alibek, Mika Vogel, Wei Sun, David Winkler, Christopher Baker, Michael Burke, and Hubertus Gloger, "Acoustic Noise Reduction in MRI Using Silent Scan: An Initial Experience," *Diagnostic and Interventional Radiology* 20 (2014): 360.
89 Mark McJury and Frank Shellock, "Auditory Noise Association with MR Procedures: A Review," *Journal of Magnetic Resonance Imaging* 12 (2000): 37.
90 Thomas Rickert, *Ambient Rhetoric: The Attunements of Rhetorical Being* (Pittsburg, PA: University of Pittsburg Press, 2013).
91 Sue Sendelbach and Marjorie Funk, "Alarm Fatigue: A Patient Safety Concern," *AACN Advanced Critical Care* 24, no. 4 (2013): 378–86.
92 Ibid., 378.
93 Bradford D. Winters, Maria M. Cyach, Christopher P. Bonafide, Xiao Hu, Avinash Konkani, Michael F. O'Connor, Jeffrey M. Rothschild et al., "Technological Distractions (Part 2): A Summary of Approaches to Manage Clinical Alarms with Intent to Reduce Alarm Fatigue," *Read Online: Critical Care Medicine| Society of Critical Care Medicine* 46, no. 1 (2018): 130–7.
94 Kierra Jones, "Alarm Fatigue a Top Patient Safety Hazard," *Canadian Medical Association Journal* 186, no. 3 (February 2014): 178; Laura Wallis, "Alarm Fatigue Linked to Patient's Death," *American Journal of Nursing* 110, no. 7 (2010): 16.
95 Ibid., para. 3.
96 *Food and Drug Administration. Manufacturer and User Device Experience (MAUDE) Database: Alarm Related Death Events 3/1/10– 6/30/10.*
97 Maria Cvach, "Monitor Alarm Fatigue: An Integrative Review," *Biomedical Instrumentation & Technology* 46, no. 4 (2012): 268–77.
98 Neda Asadi, Fatemeh Salmani, Narges Asgari, and Mahin Salmani, "Alarm Fatigue and Moral Distress in ICU Nurses in COVID-19 Pandemic," *BMC Nursing* 21, no. 1 (2022): 1–7.
99 Tamara L. Goldsby, Michael E. Goldsby, Mary McWalters, and Paul J. Mills, "Effects of Singing Bowl Sound Meditation on Mood, Tension, and Well-Being: An Observational Study," *Journal of Evidence-Based Complementary & Alternative Medicine* 22, no. 3 (2017): 401–6.

100 Adam Liptak, "Supreme Court Lets Kentucky Abortion Ultrasound Law Take Effect," *New York Times*, December 9, 2019, https://www.nytimes.com/2019/12/09/us/supreme-court-kentucky-abortion-ultrasound.html.
101 Ibid., para. 3.
102 Legislative Tracker, "Heartbeat Bans," last updated May 30, 2019, https://rewirenewsgroup.com/legislative-tracker/law-topic/heartbeat-bans.
103 Edgar, "The Rhetoric of Auscultation," 350–1.
104 Ibid., 351.
105 Dabney P. Evans and Subsasri Narasimhan, "A Narrative Analysis of Anti-Abortion Testimony and Legislative Debate Related to Georgia's Fetal 'Heartbeat' Abortion Ban," *Sexual and Reproductive Health Matters*, 28, no. 1 (2020): 218, https://doi.org/10.1080/26410397.2019.1686201.
106 Julius Hays Hess, *Premature and Congenitally Diseased Infants* (Philadelphia, PA: Lea & Febiger, 1922), 208.
107 Wikipedia, 1911, "Hearson's 'Thermostatic Nurse,'" Wikimedia Foundation. Last modified January 1, 1911. https://commons.wikimedia.org/wiki/File:EB1911_Incubators_-_Fig._14.%E2%80%94Hearson%E2%80%99s_%E2%80%9CThermostatic_Nurse%E2%80%9D.jpg.

4 Unintentional Sound and Earwitnessing in a Neonatal Intensive Care Unit[i]

In the previous two chapters, I used pan-historiography[1] to provide a panned account of rhetorically mediated sound in health and healing contexts across time. Rhetorically mediated sound provides the foundation for medico-sonic knowledge about the body. A medico-sonic knowledge of the body entails understanding and interpreting what the sounds of the body represent, diagnostically, predictively, therapeutically, and clinically. For example, Laënnec's auditory observations quite intentionally presented in *de l'auscultation médiate* as rhetorical similes and metaphors used rhetoric to systematize and catalogue heart, intestine, and lung sounds for widespread diagnostic clinical education. Or take Rice's foray into the wild at Guy's and St. Thomas' U.K. National Health Service Hospital Trust to learn cardiac auscultation and the auditory knowledge presented in the "chest rotation" that relied on "acoustic traces of bodily processes"[2] as well as rhetoric's onomatopoeia, metaphor, and simile. Either the unaided ear or a stethoscope assists intentional listening to the body's sounds to make sense of the body's condition and rely on medico-sonic knowledge to make decisions in health and healing contexts.

Rice characterized stethoscopic auscultation as "a solitary, isolating perceptual experience."[3] He explained that "This is partly because the sounds of the body are not publicly shared in the way that music played over a stereo, for instance, might be."[4] However, the content of this chapter supports my disagreement with Rice's categorization of the body's sounds in this way, especially when other health technologies are used to sonically amplify the body's sounds. In this chapter, I zoom in and focus on a particular hospital context where healthcare technologies and their sounds—powered by rhetoric—discipline bodies and instigate action. The rhetorical, sonic work of healthcare technologies and the noises they emit require *sonological competence*—the unification of "impression with cognition [making] it possible to formulate

i The current chapter was developed from "A neonatal intensive care unit (NICU) soundscape: Physiological monitors, rhetorical ventriloquism, and earwitnessing," which originally appeared in the journal *Rhetoric of Health & Medicine.*

DOI: 10.4324/9781032724416-4

and express sonic perceptions"[5]—and Michel Chion's *specialist listening*, or medico-sonic expertise, as well. In other words, in health, healing, and hospital contexts, as the previous two chapters demonstrate, sound is used as a measure to assess the body and its condition, whether as a cough or sneeze or diagnostically with an unaided ear, through auscultation mediated by a stethoscope, or therapeutically via an ultrasound, tuning fork, or MRI.

I categorize sound as either intentional or unintentional; intentional uses are diagnostic, prognostic, or therapeutic and unintentional are primarily prompted by sound as a by-product of the other three intentional diagnostic, prognostic, or therapeutic uses. The rhetorical work of unintentional sound transforms the once ineffable, internal functions of our bodies into sonic, non-discursive elements embodied in the listener. Sounds presented in medico-sonic catalogues, such as Laënnec's *de l'auscultation médiate* or cough frequencies extracted by AI using CoughSense, and amplified through healthcare technologies, such as physiological monitors and ventilators, prompt reactions and actions. Some reactions are caused in part by being without medico-sonic knowledge, then being sonically startled by alarm sounds spreading like sonic shrapnel. In health and healing contexts, unintentional, purposeless sound—or just noise—is disturbing to hearers, causing confusion, reactions, doubt, and in some cases of alarm fatigue, death.

Without the aural expertise that medico-sonic knowledge requires, the body is just uninterpretable, functional noise—breath sounds like a whistle, but what does that clinically mean? For example, Chion's classification of modes of listening as causal, semantic, or reduced demonstrate that listeners have three distinct aural purposes: determining sources (causal), interpreting messages (semantic), or characterizing sounds (reduced).[6] In particular, semantic listening functions as the mode to decipher a code, such as Morse, or interpret a message. Although Rice previously stated that listening through auscultation by stethoscope is causative—a designation I disagree with—and "reduced,"[7] medico-sonic understandings require experienced interpretation. Sound in health in healing is semantic, relying on expertise and experience—or Schaefer's sonological competence—to understand the heart's beating patterns via stethoscopic auscultation or the sounds and noises produced by physiological monitors, ventilators, and a medication dispensing machine. It also requires knowledge of how they function in a health and healing space within a hospital context. Intentional sound and unintentional noise display rhetorical power and shape care as the study in this chapter demonstrates.

I acknowledge the interconnectedness of available senses, yet when sonic activity performs as rhetorical ventriloquists—on behalf of science-based, allopathic Western biomedicine—the sonic and concatenative effects from healthcare technologies are also rhetorically-powered. Arguing from the confluence where the ineffable transforms into an influential voice and actor—powered by rhetoric—in hospital contexts, the question guiding the chapter, asks:

• what influence does unintentional sound demonstrate in a hospital context?

By acting as "earwitnesses"[8]—a field research practice described in more detail in the next chapter—who listen and attend to healthcare technologies in hospital and clinical settings, scholars can theorize how sounds shape care, send meaningful messages, and discipline bodies. More than 50 years ago, Marshall McLuhan pronounced, "Many people would be disposed to say that it was not the machine, but what one did with the machine, that was the meaning or message."[9] McLuhan's statement suggests technology as mediator for meanings or messages; however, healthcare technologies are more than mere mediators—they are influential and rhetorical actors and associated members of powerful soundscapes within hospital contexts. Physiological monitors are ubiquitous healthcare technologies we might attend to as part of soundscapes. Connected to bodies for healthcare purposes typically in hospital and other clinical environments, technologies monitor and signify health indicators or vital signs, such as heart rate, breathing or respiratory rate, blood pressure, and body temperature.

As demonstrated in the previous chapter, sound's history in health and healing is as least as long as cuneiform and hieratic recorded human history, yet its integration with technology to amplify the body's internal functions is more recent and steadier since Laënnec. Although these healthcare technologies produce multimodal, multisensory messages that seem benign or only beneficial, sonic messages from monitors contribute to a range of effects, including helpful and harmful ones. In NICU settings, for example, alarms signaling when an infant's vital signs fall out of a predetermined range have been shown to not only disrupt their sleep and cause hearing loss for infants hospitalized in NICUs,[10, 11, 12] but also contribute to nursing fatigue[13] and patient deaths.[14, 15]

Those afflicted with respiratory diseases, such as severe acute respiratory syndrome coronavirus 2 (SARS-CoV-2—the virus that causes COVID-19), often require ventilators to assist with their breathing. During the early weeks of the pandemic spreading in 2020, when healthcare systems throughout most of the world counseled and mandated people to stay home, I thought about the sonic experiences of people hospitalized with coronavirus. In hospitals, they were likely isolated, and if conscious or even unconscious, listened to the beeps of physiological monitors and whirs of ventilators, such as those described and recorded by @nurse_sushi. For some hospitals, ventilators were in short supply as global healthcare systems struggled to meet needs during the pandemic. I often thought some of the last sounds individuals who succumbed to SARS-CoV-2 infections heard were soundscapes dominated by physiological monitors and ventilators like those described by @nurse_sushi.

In the sections that follow, I provide definitions of essential terms and concepts specifically related to soundscapes. Next, prior to explaining the methodology and briefly reflecting on my own aural experience, I situate the chapter within the NICU soundscape and case study in the southwestern United States. Then I discuss the functions and effects of specific healthcare technologies that shape caretaking behaviors in this setting: physiological monitors, ventilators, and an automated medicine dispensing machine. Finally, I conclude by rhetorically uniting the history of sound in health and healing from the previous chapters with terminology to promote a sonically oriented, rhetorical theorization of sound in health, healing, and hospital contexts.

Theorizing Sonicity and Aurality in Soundscapes

In the case study presented in this chapter, I examine non-discursive, technologically produced and human interaction sounds and noises as sonic elements within a NICU's soundscape. Recall R. Murray Schafer coined and defined soundscapes as an "acoustic [or sonic] environment."[16] *Sonic elements* are those related to sounds and noises or the nature of those sounds. *Aural components* are related to the sense of hearing. Both are parts of soundscapes. An important distinction that frames understandings of soundscapes in health and healing contexts is intent or lack thereof. In other words, is the sound intentional and purposeful or not—is it noise? *Noises* are any unwanted sound; unmusical sound; any loud sound; or any disturbance in any signaling system.[17] Schafer further clarified the distinction between sounds and noises, claiming the former can transform into the unintentional noises "we have learned to ignore"[18] in soundscapes. In soundscapes, then, intentional sounds and unintentional noises intermix and produce the sonic environment, which directly influences and impacts listeners' aural, embodied experiences; shapes their actions, interactions, and reactions; and disciplines bodies.

In hospital settings such as the NICU discussed here, physiological monitors and ventilators produce *purposeful, intentional sounds* that signify important clinical events and *disruptive, unintentional noises* that distract and represent unimportant clinical events, yet also discipline bodies in the NICU. Furthermore, a third kind of healthcare technology includes a secure, automated medication dispensary machine. These machines provide measures to store and dispense controlled substances, such as opioids, and antibiotics, functioning like mobile, self-contained, secure pharmacies. And although the medication dispensing system does not produce similarly complex sounds and noises when compared with physiological monitors and ventilators, the presence of the medication dispensary machine shapes caretaking practices and interactions in NICUs, while also provoking and requiring speech that occupies the NICU's soundscape and disciplining bodily actions. For example, when a registered nurse (RN) needs to retrieve a medication from the dispensary, they must vocalize the need by asking, "Can you witness?" to any RN in the vicinity. Then, before the RN can access the medication, another RN must physically bring their body to the medication dispensary machine to witness.

Like the distinction McLuhan makes with aural intent and technology, the "acoustic environment"[19] of soundscapes are made of keynote sounds, signals, and soundmarks,[20] which can be distinguished regarding intent, purpose, and utility. Within a NICU soundscape, healthcare technologies' sounds are often intentional, serving as aural *signals* or "acoustic warning devices" that relay "elaborate codes permitting messages of considerable complexity to be transmitted to those who can interpret them."[21] In the NICU, the "elaborate codes" of the physiological monitors and ventilators are deciphered by the nurses and other healthcare clinicians who possess medico-sonic knowledge and sonological competence[22] or semantic listening[23] expertise to do so. To some—especially non-experts like me—the sounds and noises produced by some healthcare technologies are seemingly benign and probably indistinguishable from one another without medico-sonic knowledge or sonological competence. Understanding the sounds requires more than reduced listening and characterizing or describing sounds.[24] To others, like RNs, physicians, respiratory therapists, and other healthcare clinicians, these healthcare technologies can signal important healthcare events that they can clinically interpret—drawing from their medico-sonic lexicon—to act or not.

In any case, regardless of listener expertise, physiological monitors do not withhold sonic information, nor can hearing people shut out the sounds and noises with earlids. If you are hearing and within earshot, you will hear the sounds representing a body's vital signs, mediated and amplified through physiological monitors. To illustrate, think of the last time you were in a hospital, or perhaps watching, listening, or reading captioning to an episode of Grey's Anatomy, ER, Chicago Med, Offspring, Scrubs, or Nurse Jackie. The sound of these healthcare technologies are surprisingly unsophisticated, especially when compared with the advanced rhetorical and medical work they do interpreting the body's vitality. For example, physiological monitors produce messages, like the tell-tale long, sharp onomatopoeic b-e-e-e-e-e-e-p sound to indicate a person has no heart rate and that they are experiencing cardiac arrest. Usually, the b-e-e-e-e-e-e-p stimulates a flurry of activity by healthcare practitioners. However, from time to time, a connection or wire might be lost or loosened from the infant's body to the healthcare technology. For instance, I observed a parent change an infant's diaper, and in the process the heart rate rhythm patch became disconnected, causing the monitor to alarm and produce a disruptive, unimportant noise. The veteran NICU parent, though, looked at their child and remarked "he's pink," so the alarm was false. When unintentional—or unchecked—the medico-sonic presentations of bodily processes through these healthcare technologies are disrupting, unrefined, and potentially hazardous.

Physiological monitors signify heart rates, respiratory rates, blood pressure, and body temperature. Their use in healthcare settings, such as hospitals, is paramount in communicating the body's vitality when a healthcare professional is not near a patient's bedside, yet the patient's condition requires their attention. In other words, when the sense of sight is not used or available to care for patients, nurses, physicians, and other healthcare clinicians rely on physiological monitors to produce purposeful sounds they hear, then use their medico-sonic knowledge to interpret and determine what action or kind of care the infant needs from the sound's signal. As physiological monitors and ventilators populate the soundscape with sounds and noises representing embodied functions, they also amplify infants' bodies. Although these healthcare technologies provide invaluable assistance to workers (and parents) in healthcare contexts, the sonic qualities they exhibit share the crude, unsophisticated resemblance to ancient Egyptian debdeb and its use of rhetoric's onomatopoeia. Laënnec's medico-sonic rhetorical work in *de l'auscultation médiate* relied on slightly more sophisticated rhetorical devices—simile and metaphor. Yet, the cognitive work sonological competence in hospital contexts requires to interpret the onomatopoeic b-e-e-e-e-e-e-p of a heart's beat at any tempo involves all three kinds of Chion's types of listening: causal, reduced, and semantic. Healthcare clinicians determine the source of the sound (causal), the characteristics of the sound (reduced), and the sound's message or meaning (semantic)—a hefty medico-sonic cognitive demand.

Rhetorical Ventriloquism

Ventriloquism happens when a speaker utters sounds and those sounds appear to come from somewhere else. As a rhetorical concept, Cooren theorized rhetorical ventriloquism as a communicative agent defined as "the various ways by which human interactants make certain entities (collectives, procedures, policies, ideologies, etc.) speak in their name and vice versa."[25] Although Cooren does not discuss rhetorical ventriloquism primarily as embodied, he accounts for how the collectives, procedures, policies, and ideologies impact our bodies. As I am adapting rhetorical ventriloquism for a hospital setting, rhetorical ventriloquism focuses, in part, on what or who is being ventriloquized, and to what effect. It is my argument that the body's ineffability (or the sounds of the body) are rhetorically ventriloquized through health technologies and—like a ventriloquist—amplify physiological sound, yet also discipline bodies in hospitals regardless of medico-sonic knowledge.

Analogous to the rhetorical pan-historiography of sound in ancient health and healing systems from the previous chapters, in the NICU case study presented now, bodily sounds are ineffable and unable to be put into words. However, unlike ancient and modern physicians who used other rhetorical devices to develop a medico-sonic system to understand the body's sounds through onomatopoeia, metaphor, and simile, healthcare technologies in science-based, allopathic Western biomedicine today perform different work, rhetorically. When soundwaves from healthcare technologies are rhetorically considered, they sonically display and demonstrate authority and power through healthcare technologies. Healthcare technologies perform as rhetorical ventriloquists sonically adept at presenting sound as appearing from somewhere—our bodies—yet emanating from elsewhere—science-based, allopathic Western biomedicine and its technologies. Then, when these rhetorically ventriloquized soundwaves are metaphorically gathered, they generate an ensemble that sonically produces and appears as medico-sonic knowledge, simultaneously requiring interpretation and disciplining listening bodies. In this way, rhetorical ventriloquism is a materialist-feminist and phenomenological concept that re-prioritizes embodied experiences and "... [brings] the body back."[26] Alaimo's materialist-feminist concept of trans-corporeality contends "the time-space where human corporeality, in all its material fleshiness, is inseparable from 'nature' or 'environment.'"[27] As Melonçon explains, "phenomenology is a theoretical and methodological way of privileging the living and being of people,"[28] which are often "known [only] through sensory experiences."[29] When paired together, Melonçon's privileging of our living and being echoes Alaimo's trans-corporeal approach and solidifies a motivation for attending to sound—and sensory experiences—and its rhetorical power and influence in hospital contexts.

Lydia M. McDermott provides a pertinent embodied and technological example of a sonic attunement to the structure of sensory experiences.[30] McDermott suggests sonograms or ultrasounds function through a type of rhetorical ventriloquism. Extending rhetorical ventriloquism to healthcare encounters co-shaped by technologically produced sounds, she claims, "An ultrasound machine searches the contours of the womb, bouncing sound off tissue, creating a fuzzy electronic image of space: of sound."[31] Explaining her take on Cooren's rhetorical ventriloquism through the example of a sonogram's sound representing a uterus, McDermott adds that "ideals, principles, as well as organizations can communicate through a figure."[32] The NICU's healthcare technologies also use rhetorical ventriloquism; however, while McDermott's ultrasound represents a uterus, the NICU healthcare technologies I study shape healthcare attention and discipline bodies through mediated and amplified sounds and noises originating from deep within infants' sonically presented bodies—amplified for all who can hear to hear. Problematized by rhetorical ventriloquism, sonic presentation is not possible without amplification. Like McDermott's ultrasounds, the physiological monitors and ventilators derive from a body's silent process. In the case of ultrasound, a fetus's formation; and for the physiological monitors, the heart's beat, the blood's pressure, or the breath's movement. Sonic amplification of bodies requires medico-sonic knowledge, aural expertise, and a specialized blend of causal, reduced, and semantic listening[33] to understand. Recall Schafer explains this expertise as *sonological competence* or the unification of "impression with cognition [making] it possible to formulate and express sonic perceptions."[34] In other words, to aurally (and cognitively) understand the messages healthcare technologies emit, listeners must blend three listening modes, possess medico-sonic knowledge, and demonstrate sonological competence. Thus, when Chion's three listening modes are blended with sonological competence or expertise—cognitive, embodied functions—using medico-sonic knowledge, listeners decipher whether a sonic element is either a purposeful, intentional sound or a disruptive, unintentional noise.

Rhetorical ventriloquism simultaneously leverages science-based, allopathic Western biomedicine's tendency to fracture and sonically discipline bodies, operationalizes Melonçon's performative phenomenology, and enacts Alaimo's trans-corporeality, returning focus to the body, the environment, and the body's experience in the environment. Whereas there are notable exceptions, such as CAM, science-based, allopathic Western biomedicine privileges biological and physiological ways of knowing, treating, and examining bodies from what Foucault named "the medical gaze,"[35] which separates the body into its parts, functions, and conditions. I suggest that the sonic aspects of healthcare technologies produce an environment or soundscape that shapes care and caretaking, disciplines bodies, and provides biomedical representations of bodies within hospital contexts. In the process, while their sounds encourage initial attention to technologies rather than bodies, trans-corporeal, phenomenological understandings of rhetorical ventriloquism subsequently re-focus attention on bodies, on senses, and on healthcare and clinical settings as sonic sites. Accordingly, rhetorical ventriloquism offers a novel, productive framework for understanding soundscapes in health and medical contexts and further extends the concept of medico-sonic knowledge.

The NICU Ward: Aurality in Critical Care Context

The participants for this chapter's case study were chosen using a purposeful sampling technique to identify participants with specific characteristics.[36] I sought participants who were willing to consent to participate in my study, who spoke English, and who were nurses and parents or other legal caregivers of infants hospitalized in a NICU in the southwestern United States. I observed participants—nurses, parents, and other legal caregivers—from about twenty feet or 6 meters away to provide physical space and privacy between the participants and myself. Mostly, my sight lines were unobstructed during observations. The infants were in relatively stable conditions; in other words, the nursing and medical staff deemed these infants not in immediate danger of destabilizing in life-threatening ways.[ii] Before commencing my study, I obtained Institutional Review Board[iii] (IRB) approvals from the university and the university's medical school and NICU's affiliated hospital. After participants ($n = 20$) consented, I observed parents ($n = 8$), other legal caregivers ($n = 2$), and nurses ($n = 10$); if available and still willing, I interviewed participants ($n = 13$), including nurses ($n = 9$) and parents ($n = 4$), after observations. All observations occurred in the NICU, primarily in one nursery with seven infants. I interviewed participants in private and semi-private spaces within the NICU and hospital. For example, I interviewed several parents in a small, private waiting room with two couches and a door outside of the secure NICU. However, in instances when nurses were unable to leave the NICU, I Interviewed them in various, semi-private locations, such as an empty pod or near an infant's bedside. The interviews were digitally audio recorded and later transcribed—an integral, sonic process that emphasized the NICU soundscape for me in surprising ways.

Joshua Gunn previously noted the emotionally "punishing affects" of listening to recorded speech.[37] I transcribed by listening to the digitally recorded participant interviews through earphones. I did not experience the punitive impact Gunn describes; however, I markedly noticed healthcare technologies and their performance as sonic shrapnel in the background of interviews. As the physiological monitors frequently issued alarms at decibels higher than normal spoken conversation, I had to remove the earphones and take periodic breaks. It was during transcription I decided to examine sound more closely.

Specifically, as part of a larger, multi-site study, the original research questions I aimed to answer included: What patient information is communicated to those who are legally responsible for neonates—namely parents or foster parents, grandparents, and/or social workers—in NICUs? Who or what communicates this information, how, and when? After I identified how the healthcare

---

ii Although some infants are hospitalized in NICUs because they are extremely premature or sick with life-threatening conditions, some infants are housed in NICUs because of the unfortunate conditions associated with being born too early or sick (morbidity). Further, a neonatal nurse—at most hospitals in the United States—attends higher risk deliveries, such as cesarean sections, and when there are known complications, such as multiple births, like twins or triplets. Regardless, highly specialized neonatal nurses are clinically equipped to care for infants who may need to grow before they can be discharged because they were born too early or sick. Labor and delivery nurses—skilled at helping pregnant people labor and deliver infants—are trained to care and attend deliveries for normal births and infants that do not require specialized care. Neonatal nurses, however, are skilled to take care and attend deliveries for a range of infants born too early or sick with various conditions associated with being born too early or sick. It was understood and agreed upon that if an infant destabilized, I would immediately stop observing and remove myself from the immediate vicinity.

iii The study was approved by University and University Health Sciences institutional review boards—two human ethics review committees.

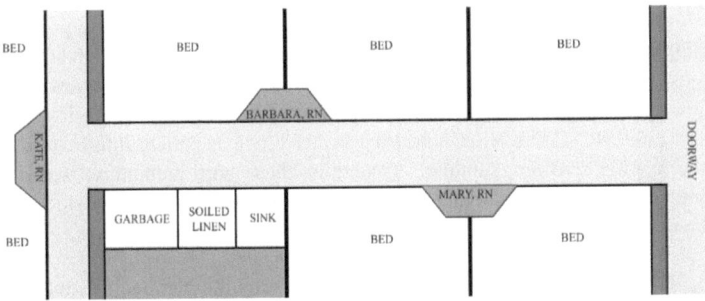

Figure 4.1 Open-bay layout of one of the three NICU nurseries.

technologies were sending messages as part of the NICU's soundscape, I expanded my questions to include "What responses are the sounds prompting and to what a/effects?" The southwestern NICU has been described as an advanced healthcare space that incorporates ambient lighting and technologies to reduce sound, such as cushioned, noise dampening floor tiles and sound-absorbing ceiling tiles. The NICU is a level IV NICU; it provides the highest level of clinical care for critical infants, including heart and lung bypasses through two extracorporeal membrane oxygenation (ECMO) beds. Additionally, the NICU is a regional transport center that can hold nearly 40 infants in its three larger nurseries connected by hallways, inclusive of one unit.

As seen in Figure 4.1, the layout of these NICU nurseries is an open-bay design. Parents and other legal caregivers pull curtains closed for privacy. For example, privacy curtains are shut if a parent is breast or chest feeding their infant; however, those curtains are not soundproof. The NICU soundscape easily permeates throughout the open-bay pod and unit and through privacy curtains. From behind the curtains, conversations were heard between parents and other legal caregivers, as well as private conversations between physicians, nurses, and parents. For instance, I unintentionally overheard a private conversation between a physician and an infant's parent about circumcising the infant prior to discharge.

Rest time and growing time are essential for neonates in NICUs. To that end, in addition to common policies regarding patient visiting hours, the NICU had two policies—as RN Kate[iv] described—to cluster infant care ("touch time") and provide quiet time ("siesta time") for sleeping and growing. As stated on a sign at the NICU entrance, during siesta time from 1:30 pm to 3:00 pm, the NICU must be quiet to mimic the ideal sound environment for sleeping infants. The importance of controlling sound levels is apparent in the NICU's "siesta time" policy, which shapes caretaking practices and impacts actions in the NICU.

---

iv All names are pseudonyms.

Quiet time policies like "siesta time" show an awareness of the importance of quiet and, in turn, sound to health, healing, and growing for premature and sick infants in the NICU. In fact, hearing healthcare is addressed for newborns. For example, each NICU infant has a hearing screening prior to discharge from the NICU. The NICU's hearing center provides patient information on the hearing screening, stating: "Generally, those born premature, requiring intensive care, or those with a family history of hearing loss are considered to be at high risk for hearing loss." Further, the hearing center explains:

> Even with passing [hearing screening] results the National Institutes of Health, supported by the American Academy of Pediatrics, recommends a three month audiological re-evaluation for infants who were treated in the NICU and six month re-evaluation for all other babies to rule out the development of a progressive hearing loss or one that is fluctuating in nature due to recurrent middle ear problems.

Clearly, NICUs recognize hearing loss as a common issue for neonates, which further suggests their hearing should be shielded from unnecessary noises. As I pointed out in previous chapters, researchers identified and explored the phenomenon of "alarm fatigue" or when nurses and other health clinicians are "… exposed to an excessive number of alarms, which can result in desensitization to alarms and missed alarms"[38] and cause missed important, clinical alarms.

It is evident that important, clinical sounds and unimportant, distracting noises produce a soundscape with the power to shape care, caretaking practices, and discipline bodies. Foucault theorized such bodily disciplining in *Discipline and Punish*. With the addition of sound—a "disciplinary method"[39]—in hospital contexts, much like in elementary schools, hearing bodies are trained to provide their attention "at the first sound of the bell."[40] He continues by theorizing a student's action by describing it as "whenever a good pupil hears the noise of the signal, he will imagine that he is hearing the voice of the teacher or rather the voice of God himself calling him by name."[41] In such fantastically active sonic contexts as hospitals, does sound rhetorically function as science-based, allopathic Western biomedicine? Is there ever quiet in a NICU (or anywhere within a hospital unit) when such healthcare technologies are used? In other words, as the latter portion of the previous chapter demonstrates, since sound functions as an intentional mainstay in health and healing contexts, what rhetorical power can it wield?

NICU Soundscape Healthcare Technologies: Physiological Monitors, Ventilators, and the Automated Medication Dispensing System

Although there are many kinds of healthcare technologies occupying hospital and clinical settings, during my observations and interviews the physiological monitors, ventilators, and an automated medication dispensing system most frequently emitted sound and demanded attention. As such, these three health-care technologies—and primarily the physiological monitors—most obviously suggested how technologically produced and amplified sounds shaped the care of the neonates in the NICU and worked as rhetorical ventriloquists for science-based, allopathic Western biomedicine. However, the physiological monitors and ventilators affected the soundscape differently than the automated medication dispensing system. For example, acting as an earwitness in the NICU, I realized the physiological monitors and ventilators directly made noises and sounds; however, the automated medication dispensing system indirectly required speech sounds or vocalization via a hospital policy regulating its use. Regardless, these three healthcare technologies contributed to the NICU soundscape, shaped caretaking practices, and disciplined the bodies of those I observed within this hospital context.

Physiological Monitors

Acting as an earwitness when entering the NICU, I noticed the soundscape is dominated by physiological monitors that signal when infant vital signs fall outside predetermined ranges and voices talking about various care-related topics. The vital signs physiological monitors gauge are heart rate, respiratory rate, blood pressure, and body temperature. Additionally, a separate probe—typically placed around an infant's foot—reports blood oxygen saturation or pulse oximetry (pulse ox). Blood oxygen saturation—with a separate pulse ox lead that plugs into the physiological monitor—relays its information through the physiological monitor both visually and aurally. For example, because an infant's predetermined range for acceptable blood oxygen saturation is, say, 92–95%, blood oxygen saturation above or below that range triggers the monitor's alarm (and shows as a visual blinking number) to alert all who can hear within earshot or see nearby. In an intensive care unit, simultaneously (often continuously) sounding alarms throughout the unit are common, as noted when I transcribed the digitally recorded interviews with participants.

The physiological monitors that sonically alert nurses about an infant's vital statistics (in the NICU or any hospital unit) are the hallmark noisemakers or "soundmarks"[42] in biomedical healthcare. Schafer defines *soundmarks* as the "community sound which is unique or possesses qualities which make it specially regarded or noticed by the people in that community,"[43] such as those heard or read in closed captioning when viewing or listening to an episode of Grey's Anatomy or Chicago Med. The onomatopoeiac ping-ding-ding-ding of physiological monitors are loud, yet become louder if the "silence" button is not pressed (or the infant vital sign causing the alarm remains outside the predetermined range). Since the alarming is nearly incessant, the healthcare technologies' sounds and noises consistently and perpetually shape care and discipline bodies in NICU contexts and act as rhetorical ventriloquists for

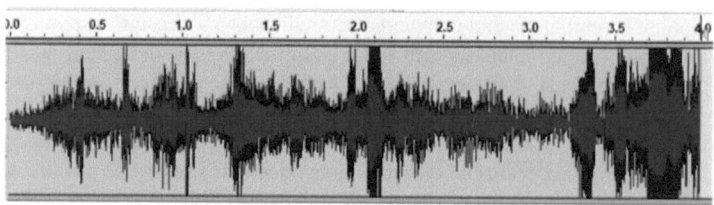

Figure 4.2 Four-second excerpt waveform of sound file 3: infant crying. There is an infant crying punctuating (2.1 and 3.3 seconds–end) the excerpt.

science-based, allopathic Western biomedicine and its priorities—treating symptoms and diseases with drugs, interventions, and operations and monitoring the body with healthcare technologies that imitate and amplify the heart's beat, the blood's pressure, or the breath's movement.

I accidentally and unintentionally contributed noise to the NICU soundscape. I did not initially understand the impact of sounds and noises in the NICU. However, once I began to transcribe the interviews, my aural sense was unpleasantly heightened. The transcription of one interview—with RN Mary—was especially telling. During the interview, Mary and I sat near her workstation in the nursery. In sound files 1 and 2,[v] I edit around voices to protect privacy and anonymity and focus on the physiological monitor alarms. As I transcribed the interview, I realized that the ding-ding-ding-dings and beep-beep-beep-beeps peppered the entire duration of the interview. In keeping with Schafer's sonological competence—or appropriately hearing and cognitively processing sounds—most of the alarming physiological monitors did not merit a nurse's attention. However, at one point, Kate walked through the unit toward what seemed to me (a non-expert without sonological competence) another benign, ignorable alarm. However, as Kate walked swiftly and passed by me and Mary, she stated, "I got it [the infant and the alarm]." As noted elsewhere,[44] to non-expert listeners alarming monitor's purposeful sounds and disruptive noises are virtually indistinguishable; in contrast, the NICU nurse could semantically listen, then competently interpret the alarms as clinical messages integral to infant care.

In sound files 1 and 2, I provide a sampling of two physiological alarm signals and clinical messages. For comparison, in sound file 3, I include a four-second snippet of the beginning of my interview with RN Mary. In the audio, I thank her for taking the time to be interviewed and state my appreciation for her participation. Further, an infant is heard crying throughout the four seconds, and there are no physiological monitors sounding. In Figure 4.2,

v   The audio files can be accessed via the online Routledge Resource Centre https://resourcecentre. routledge.com/books/9781032724379.

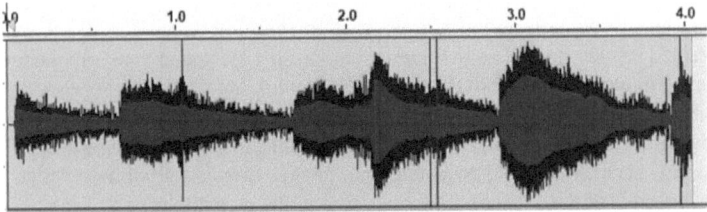

Figure 4.3 Four-second excerpt waveform of sound file 1.

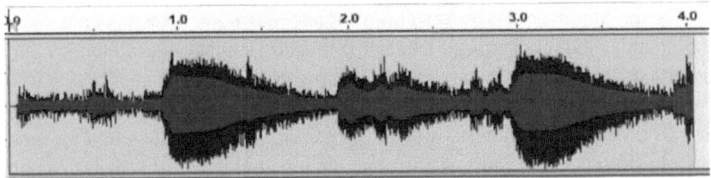

Figure 4.4 Four-second excerpt waveform of sound file 2.

I supply a visual representation of sound: a waveform of sound file 3. And in Figures 4.3 and 4.4, I present waveforms of sound files 1 and 2, respectively.

A *waveform* shows the shape of sound; the "materiality of sound."[45] The entirety of each waveform visually represents the intensity of the sounds and noises in the excerpts. The waveforms (Figures 4.3 and 4.4) reveal the visual representations of two important sonic elements: the NICU soundscape and the visualized, synchretic[46] complexity of the soundscape—a visual manifestation and representation of rhetorical ventriloquism. In the waveforms, the darkest areas farther from the waveform's horizontal midline represent more intense sounds and noises.[vi] In Figure 4.2, the infant's cry can be seen most clearly at the end of the waveform (3.3 seconds–end). After listening to sound file 3 and seeing the waveform show the shape of the sounds, bursts of noises and sounds are heard/seen. When considered alongside Linden Gledhill's image of sound[47] (displayed opposite the title page), sound's symmetry and sense demonstrates how sound appears focused and intentional even if not immediately evident in waveforms.

Physiological monitor noises and sounds result in a sonically sustained soundscape with sound and sound waves present at most times. Additionally, each of the four-second clips were intentionally curated to isolate NICU

---

vi Physics is outside the scope of my expertise; however, the punctuated sounds—the acoustical discomfort I experienced transcribing the interviews—can be described as transient. In physics terminology, "A transient is a sudden and brief burst of acoustic energy, for example a gunshot, the snap when you break a branch, a handclap. Transients occur in speech as the plosive releases of stop consonants" (https://swphonetics.com/praat/tutorials/understanding-waveforms/#diagram).

sounds and noises and visually present rhetorical ventriloquism. Further, it was not uncommon during my observations and interviews for all the ex-cerpted sounds and noises to intermix and occupy the soundscape simultane-ously. In other words, both the purposeful sounds and disruptive noises—the transient tones—of physiological monitors and human voices talking and cry-ing within the NICU soundscape are synchronous. In any critical care hospital context such as a NICU, the soundscape shapes care and disciplines bodies, irrespective of the value of the sonic signal or the expertise (that is, sonologi-cal competence) of the listener or earwitness and their mode of listening.

Distractingly, then, as the physiological monitors perform as rhetorical ventriloquists, separating bodies from their vital functions, these infants' heartbeats, blood pressures, respiration rates, and pulse oxes become com-plex, punctuated, competing tones with the body's silent vital functions and the infants themselves. In the process, nursing and caretaking attention moves from the physical body to healthcare technology's sounds and noises, which can be distracting to nurses, as well as parents and other legal caregivers. The physiological monitors amplify the body's vitality (or lack thereof) with marked, and in some cases, incessant transient alarms, which direct attention away from the body and to the healthcare technology. And although these alarms can signal important clinical events, they also falsely alarm for unim-portant ones. For instance, when a parent changing her child's diaper heard an alarm sound and remarked about the "pink" infant and ignored the alarming monitor. Also, I observed a parent and grandparent (and later, just the grand-parent) move to an infant's bedside when an alarm sounded repeatedly. Later, when I interviewed the infant's nurse, RN Kate, about that movement and the conversation with the parent and grandparent that followed, she explained,

> They were just asking me if she was okay, and I was just saying she's fine. I was just explaining to them that she's a preemie [premature baby] and a lot of time they have those issues with the apneas and bradycardia [shallow breathing and slowed heartbeat; …]

In that same interview with Kate, she confirmed that part of the conversa-tion with the parent and grandparent included potentially sending the infant home on a monitor due to the child's apnea and bradycardia; I had heard the same conversation during observation of the parent, grandparent, and Kate. I also noted that Kate remarked to the parent, "I know it's scary" after talk-ing about the at-home monitor possibility. And it is scary considering the aural sensuous training non-experts receive in NICUs which might not pro-vide opportunities to semantically listen to alarms to learn how to distinguish between important and unimportant clinical events—like the parent who re-marked about her "pink" infant and ignored the alarm.

A few bedsides away, two new parents received information about a Peripher-ally Inserted Central Catheter (PICC) for their infant from their infant's nurse,

Barbara. Prior to inserting a PICC line, parents must provide their written consent. As Barbara explained the PICC line procedure, one parent was markedly distracted by the infant's frequently alarming monitor. During the consent process, the infant's monitor sounded for unimportant clinical events; yet no doubt due to an expertise for Chion's modes of listening and sonological competence, Barbara was not distracted and kept focused on explaining the PICC consent process to the new parents. During observations, in several other instances while nurses were charting on computers or completing nursing notes about patients, I recorded in my double-entry field notes that alarms were sounding. For example, an alarm went off at an infant's bedside, and I immediately looked to Mary who was charting. Due to her sonological competence gained through blended modes of listening, she was not distracted by the noise in a noticeable way as she kept working and "clicking ... her mouse." Her response to the alarm noise—she did not move to the infant's bedside—suggested she was familiar with the kind of noise and knew it to be unimportant noise; however, unlike the parent during the PICC line consent process with Barbara or the parent and grandparent regarding the at-home monitor, Mary possessed listening mode expertise and sonological competence, so she knew how to respond to sonic cues from healthcare technologies.

Disruptive noises did not signal vitally important clinical events. If they had, nurses would have attended to the alarms and the infants. In fact, the monitors contributed noise to the NICU soundscape and sent a message to the parent and grandparent—a misunderstood message, no doubt, due to lack of sonological competence and unrefined semantic listening, which likely prompted Kate to remark, "I know it's scary." For the new parents receiving information to consent to the PICC line, the alarm's noises distracted one parent and perhaps impacted their understanding of the PICC insertion procedure. As these examples show, just as physiological monitors helpfully amplify the body's processes and vital functions, they also misconstrue the body's vitality, unhelpfully and distractingly ventriloquize, and demand and discipline attention.

Whether for an important or unimportant clinical event, the alarming physiological monitors demand attention and shape care. And when acting as an earwitness in a soundscape, the sonic becomes embodied in the aural, helping to make sense of participant actions. Acting as an earwitness in the NICU, I noticed the physiological monitors consistently alarmed and noted that some alarms required a noticeable response while others did not. Evidently, physiological monitors shape caretaking behaviors for parents, other legal caregivers, and nurses, as well as require the sonological competence and semantic listening of the listener or earwitness.

Ventilators

Ventilators are another prominent source of sounds in NICUs. If an infant needs assistance with breathing, they can be placed on one of many kinds of ventilation. For example, Continuous Positive Airway Pressure (CPAP)

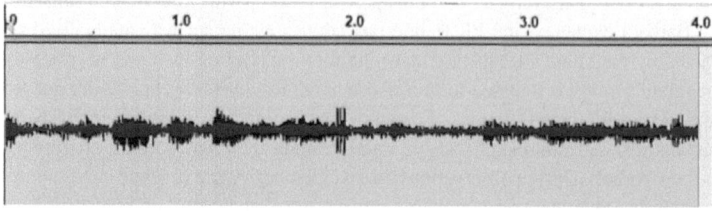

Figure 4.5 Four-second excerpt waveform of sound file 4: high frequency oscillating ventilator (HFOV) with human voice.

or Bilevel Positive Airway Pressure (BiPAP) ventilation therapies and mechanical and high frequency respiratory ventilation are assistive respiratory therapies. At one point when an alarm sounded, it woke an infant with CPAP, which was making a steady, shhhhh-like sound. In response to the alarm, the infant put their hands to the CPAP prongs. Kate explained, "… sometimes if the CPAP slips out of the nose, it can … just come out a little bit, [and] it can cause the baby to have an apnea or a desat[uration] or have a brady[cardia]." If the CPAP prongs slip out, or an infant removes them, an alarm sounds. Thus, these respiratory aids create purposeful sounds and disruptive noises. For example, a high frequency oscillating ventilator (HFOV) can be heard in sound file 4, and its waveform can be seen in Figure 4.5. Comparable to Bivens et al.[48] and an interview with a nurse, Cassie, and the noises of the HFOV, these machines necessarily assist infant breathing, shape care, and discipline bodies. Like the sound of a steam locomotive's engine, HFOV's sounds are incessant and steady as they work to assist breathing.

The NICU soundscape includes purposeful sounds for important clinical events, such as the alarms signaling before Kate exclaimed, "I got it," and disruptive noises—the ignored alarms dismissed as unimportant. Regardless of sonic importance, the soundscape easily permeates the entirety of the NICU and its pods, shaping the care of these neonates and disciplining bodies within them. Depending on acuity or criticality of the infants, as well as state laws, an RN might care for more than three NICU infants at a time. If one infant is being cared for and an alarm signals for another infant, the nurse must safely stop caring for one infant to move on to the next. Although nurses are assigned to care for infants, often they must assist each other. For example, Barbara remarked about the design of the NICU and needing help from other nurses:

> Like you know for the call lights. The call light system. […] there's nobody in here because they're in here helping you and something is going on with another baby. Well, guess what? Nobody's gonna know until this alarm starts beeping louder and louder.

Barbara noted alarms become louder and louder if not switched off or silenced. During my observations and earwitnessing, I saw and heard nurses silence the alarms before attending to infants—a visual and sonic signal to other nurses acknowledging physiological or ventilator alarms, which shapes infant care by limiting the personalized time nurses spend physically attending infants and disciplining and directing caretaking actions. In fact, throughout observations and as noted in the interview with Barbara, healthcare technologies were typically attended before infants, and if not, the "alarm starts beeping louder and louder," which is like @nurse_sushi's narrative TikTok video. Ventilators demand immediate attention and continue to alarm—regardless of importance—until attended to or the reason for the alarm resolves. In the process, ventilators and their alarms provide disciplining sounds, act as rhetorical ventriloquists, direct caretaking practices, and shape care.

Automated Medication Dispensing System

When retrieving medication using the secure, automated medicine dispensary (Pyxis MedStation™), nurses aurally "witness" other nurses to promote patient safety before accessing and administering medications. As TikTok user @beautifulnursing pointed out with the HICKOP [Heparin, Insulin, Chemotherapy, Potassium (periodic table abbreviation, K), Opioids, and Pediatric/neonate][49] mnemonic for medications needing verification by a second nurse, the "P" in HICKOP stands for "Pediatric/neonate." Consistently, and almost hourly, I heard RNs ask, "can you witness?" to other RNs, which was the question prompting medication verification. For example, Kate showed Diane two syringes filled with medication. Kate sought to have Diane "witness" or verify the correct patient's name and medication dose. To initiate the medication verification procedure, Kate asked Diane, "can you witness me?" Another time, Kate said to Mary, "caffeine [to stimulate infant breathing during apnea and bradycardia spells] check for bed six." Although caffeine is not a narcotic or controlled medication, checking all medications decreases the likelihood of administering incorrect medications or doses and initiates speech sounds. During the interview with Mary, I asked her about administering a controlled medication—an instance requiring another RN to witness. I asked, "say you have to get phenobarb[ital] for a baby, what do you have to do?"

> Mary: I have to make sure that I know how much I'm giving, and I have to check my order [from the physician], which usually, you know [...] how much a good range is; you have to [...] walk to the Pyxis (is where we keep our meds is this machine called Pyxis). [...] And it's in the med room or whatever, and so you go in there, and you have to bring someone

to witness with you; you have to type in [your code], and you have to pick out the med and the name and you have to get someone to sign into the Pyxis as well before you can get in because it's a narcotic, and then you have to […] go to the bedside […] and […] pull it out and to make sure it's the right amount so you have to calculate how much […] you have to get it and you have to check it again to make sure that it's the right amount, and then you can give it.

Any time a controlled medication, such as a narcotic like phenobarbital or morphine, is ordered for an infant, a nurse "witness" must be present before the other nurse can access and administer the medication. As Mary described, first the physician's order for the medication and dose for a particular patient must be confirmed; second, the RN must find someone to "witness" and verify the medication and infant name at the Pyxis medication machine. Mary further explained "with babies, it's like such a small amount [of medication …] if you mess it up, you can do so much damage; […] since I've been in NICU, we've always double checked like every med[ication]."

Additionally, before an infant is given expressed chest or breast milk (EBM), for a feeding by mouth (PO), gavage tube through the mouth (OG), or gavage tube through the nose (NG), an RN must verify that the labelled syringe or bottle of EBM was expressed or pumped by the infant's parent. In other words, for every infant who is not fed at chest or breast or with formula, an RN must ask "can you witness?" to another RN. Consequently, an RN caring for an infant who has medications and EBM for feedings every three hours might ask "can you witness?" eight to ten times every twenty-four hours for just one infant. Cooren argues rhetorical ventriloquists force people to speak for policies and procedures (and vice versa). Although queries to witness and verify medications are important procedures for medication safety and witnessing policies aim to protect infants, the speech sounds of witnessing related to the automated medication dispensing system act as rhetorical ventriloquists and discipline bodies to behave on behalf of policies and procedures. For example, pulling in a second nurse for a medication check temporarily removes that nurse from the care of another infant, disciplines nursing behavior and actions, and shapes the caretaking practices of both nurses and the care received by infants.

Earwitnessing, Shaping Care, and Sensuous Training and Disciplining

Amplifying sounds, healthcare technologies produce purposeful, intentional sounds and unimportant, distracting noises. Sounds and noises produce healthcare soundscapes that showcases and harnesses science-based, allopathic Western biomedicine through rhetorically-powered sound and discipline bodies in hospital contexts. Hospital policies and practices contribute to contexts requiring quiet ("siesta time") and speech (responding to medication safety and witnessing policies) prior to accessing and administering medications. Sound-producing healthcare technologies discipline bodies and shape care and caretaking in the NICU. Physiological monitors and ventilators effectively perform as rhetorical ventriloquists—where physiological monitors speak and sound for infants in a soundscape where sounds and noises appear to stand in for bodies and their physiologies, while the healthcare technologies speak and sound for those bodies. In certain instances, like when Kate stated, "I got it," the physiological monitors signal important clinical events integral to address for the health and vitality of the infant; however, in other occurrences, like when I interviewed Mary and heard several alarms in sound files 1 and 2, the alarms produce disruptive noise and do not signal important clinical events.

Elsewhere in work about multi-sensorial, layered health literacies, I included an example of the biomedicalization of an infant's sneeze.[50] In a NICU, a sleeping infant sneezed, causing an alarm to signal and produce a noise, which in turn woke the infant. The physiological monitoring of the infant's vital statistics provided a biomedical interpretation of the body and its function—the sonically and rhetorically-powered, biomedical gaze. Whether important, purposeful sounds or unimportant, disruptive noises, the soundscape is occupied by these signals, which in turn discipline bodies in hospital contexts. As I point out elsewhere, "all alarms cause alarm,"[51] which sends messages suggesting the listener or earwitness react and act, regardless of sonological competence. When parents or other legal caregivers without nursing or medical expertise (or sonological competencies, such as the parent who remarked their infant was "pink") are present in NICUs, alarms result in conflicting messages. Through semantic listening, listeners want the sound to have meaning. It is likely non-clinicians know the sounds originate from infants' bodies, which means the source of the sound—causal listening—is known. With alarms and other sonic signals, our bodies are prepared to be disciplined and behave accordingly. However, when the meaning is unknown or indecipherable—and reduced and semantic listening not possible—understandably, it is troubling and confusing. It is comparable to walking into an office building and the smoke alarms, carbon monoxide detectors, elevator alarms, and telephones all sound, alarm, or ring simultaneously as people go about their daily work. If a delivery person arrives and they are incapable of semantic listening and thus sonological competence, they might not realize why one employee responds to the tenth time a phone rings, but not the previous nine times.

Mixed messages confuse hearers and earwitnesses in NICU spaces and have been shown to negatively impact nursing care through "alarm fatigue," such as the case for @nurse_sushi,[52] as well as the hearing health of infants hospitalized in NICUs. Alarm fatigue causes nurses to miss important, clinical alarms[53] and alarm fatigue negatively influences nursing care and focus.[54]

A systematic review about the impact of alarm fatigue on the nurses in intensive care units (ICU) reported "Alarm fatigue may have serious consequences, both for patients and for nursing personnel"[55] and patient care is adversely influenced by alarm fatigue.[56] ICU nurses thought physiological monitors and their alarm sounds were burdensome, often incessant,[57] and interfere with patient care,[58,59] which also reduces their trust in these technologies.[60] @nurse_sushi[61] also commented on the omnipresent or "continuous wave"[62] of ICU physiological alarms for patients infected with the SARS-CoV-2 virus or COVID-19 disease, expressing "Alarm fatigue is high these days."

Unfortunately, sonic sensory overload is not the only problem; in extreme cases, alarm fatigue has led to patient deaths.[63,64] Kierra Jones in "Alarm Fatigue a Top Patient Safety Hazard" cites a FDA report of "566 alarm-related deaths between 2005 and 2008."[65] Jones noted that in one intensive care unit, more than 700 alarms sounded for each bed or person.[66] If nurses and infants are negatively impacted by NICU soundscapes and alarming physiological monitors, it follows that parents and other legal caregivers are deleteriously affected, too. For example, when alarms are not responded to, families can lose confidence and trust in clinical staff.[67] In hospital contexts, alarm sounds discipline bodies to behave in response. In other words, the "all alarms cause alarm" sends an imprecise message to parents and other legal caregivers that they must simultaneously hear and potentially misunderstand, while also expecting clinicians with sonological competencies to act upon. When clinicians behave with "no or delayed response" to alarms, it diminishes trust placed on clinicians who care for family members.[68]

Cooren's definition of rhetorical ventriloquism identifies collectives, procedures, and policies as items where people "speak in their name and vice versa."[69] Applied in hospital contexts, rhetorical ventriloquism is evident through healthcare technologies speaking sonically for a body's vitality. In addition to their life-saving capabilities, physiological monitors and ventilators function as rhetorical ventriloquists for these bodies, shaping their care, disciplining bodies, and influencing healthcare clinician caretaking. With both critical signals of the body's vitality and false alarms, the NICU soundscape is aurally tagged with internal physiological processes, performing as rhetorical ventriloquists and drawing from and reinforcing the disciplinary power of the hospital and its policies. Physiological processes are amplified to reveal synchretic representations of what would—without healthcare technologies—be silent and wholly occurring inside infant bodies; yet the sounds and noises eventually redirect the medical gaze back to infants in particular ways and reinforce certain caretaking behaviors. Meanwhile, parents and other legal caretakers are also disciplined and sonically trained in the critical care hospital environment.

Anne Frances Wysocki's "sensuous training" concept posits that "our sensuous perceptions of the world do not just happen 'naturally' but come to their shape in our varying, complex, and socially embedded environments."[70]

Chion's modes of listening show—regardless of our sensuous training or perceptions—certain kinds of listening are needed to determine sources of sound (causal), characterize sounds (reduced), and interpret messages from sound (semantic).[71] His modes of listening are supported in medical and nursing education, such in studies by Rice[72] and Harris and Van Drie,[73] where novice and student clinicians are taught how to listen to the body—via medico-sonic methods—with the help of rhetorical devices.

Hearing bodies and earwitnesses are trained to provide their attention "at the first sound of the bell"[74] or in hospital contexts, alarms. In NICU environments where healthcare technologies perpetually signal to experts and non-experts alike, the sensuous training has been shown to cause intermittent attention, alarm fatigue, sleep disruption, and hearing loss to listeners. The sonic shrapnel that populates hospital soundscapes continues to be worrisome. Without intentional sensory training for non-experts coupled with other methods to dampen noise and make important clinical sounds more meaningful for all, such problems likely persist. How are parents and other legal caregivers able to become sonologically competent in a healthcare environment where rhetorically ventriloquized sonic messages are amplified consistently, yet perhaps randomly? How can semantic listening be taught? Eventually and ideally, parents and other legal caregivers take their infants home. And in certain instances, like the infant referenced earlier who would likely be discharged with an at-home monitor, if the parents' sonic, sensuous exposures provided no distinction between important and unimportant clinical events and their sounds, what kind of hearing training and medico-sonic competence can they draw upon to care for their own child? Further, if parents and other legal caregivers learn to depend on physiological monitors to signal when their infants need attention (from previous sonic sensuous exposure, training, and discipline), does that reliance and confusion reinforce biomedical ways of knowing and disciplining bodies outside clinical settings? In various ways, then, parents and other legal caregivers face challenges surrounding sonic competence and semantic listening once infants go home.

During nearly 100 hours of observations in NICUs in the United States (and part of the larger study in Denmark), whenever I witnessed nurses, parents, and other legal caregivers at infant bedsides when alarms sounded, invariably nurses instructed parents to look at their infants, like the parent who remarked their infant was "pink" in color. For example, if an alarm sounded and the monitor showed a crying infant without a heart rate, then it was a false alarm. Parents and other legal caregivers could ascertain similarly by looking at the infant. However, in certain instances, the biomedical gaze forces those tasked with caring for these infants to first look to an alarming physiological monitor, then to the child—a message rhetorically vocalized and ventriloquized from discipline and sensuous training then corrected by looking away from biomedicine and back to the body. Wysocki declares, "without our bodies—our sensing abilities—we do not have a world; we have the world we do because we have our particular senses and experiences."[75] Fully attending to sounds in hospital contexts recognizes how healthcare technologies spur action, require attention, shape experiences, and discipline hearing and deaf bodies alike.

Notes

1 Debra Hawhee and Christa J. Olson, "Pan-historiography: The Challenges of Writing History across Time and Space," in *Theorizing Histories of Rhetoric*, ed. Michelle Ballif (Carbondale, IL: Southern Illinois University Press, 2013), 90–105.
2 Rice, Tom, "Learning to Listen: Auscultation and the Transmission of Auditory Knowledge," *Journal of the Royal Anthropological Institute* 16 (2010): S44.
3 Ibid., S51.
4 Ibid., S51.
5 F. Murray Schafer, *The Soundscape: Our Sonic Environment and the Tuning of the World* (Rochester, VT: Destiny Books, 1977/1994), 274.
6 Chion, Michel, "The Three Listening Modes," *The Sound Studies Reader*, ed. Jonathan Sterne (New York: Routledge, 2012), 48–53.
7 Ibid.
8 Schafer, *The Soundscape*, 272.
9 Marshall McLuhan, *Understanding Media: The Extensions of Man* (Cambridge, MA: MIT Press, 1964/1994), 7.
10 Charlene Krueger, Elan Horesh, and Brian Adam Crossland. "Safe Sound Exposure in the Fetus and Preterm Infant." *Journal of Obstetric, Gynecologic & Neonatal Nursing* 41, no. 2 (2012): 166–70.
11 Roberto Antonucci, Annalisa Porcella, and Vassilios Fanos, "The Infant Incubator in the Neonatal Intensive Care Unit: Unresolved Issues and Future Developments." *Journal of Perinatal Medicine*, 37 no. 6 (2009): 587–98.
12 Hsin-Li Chen, Chao-Huei Chen, Chih-Chao Wu, Hsiu-Jung Huang, Teh-Ming Wang, and Chia-Chi Hsu, "The Influence of Neonatal Intensive Care Unit Design on Sound Level," *Pediatrics & Neonatology* 50 no. 6 (2009): 270–4.
13 Sue Sendelbach and Marjorie Funk, "Alarm Fatigue: A Patient Safety Concern," *AACN Advanced Critical Care*, 24, no. 4 (2013): 378–86.
14 Kierra Jones. "Alarm Fatigue a Top Patient Safety Hazard." *CMAJ: Canadian Medical Association Journal*, vol. 186 no. 3 (2014), 178.
15 Laura Wallis, "Alarm Fatigue Linked to Patient's Death," *AJN: The American Journal of Nursing* 110, no. 7 (2010): 16.
16 Schafer, *The Soundscape*, 7.
17 Ibid., 273.
18 Ibid., 4.
19 Ibid., 7.
20 Ibid., 9.
21 Ibid., 10.
22 Ibid., 274.
23 Chion, "The Three Listening Modes," 48.
24 Ibid.
25 François Cooren, "The Selection of Agency as a Rhetorical Device: Opening up the Scene of Dialogue through Ventriloquism," *Dialogue and Rhetoric* (2008): 23–24.
26 Lisa Melonçon, "Bringing the Body Back through Performative Phenomenology," in *Methodologies for the Rhetoric of Health & Medicine*, eds. Lisa Melonçon and J. Blake Scott (New York: Routledge: 2018), 100.

27 Stacy Alaimo, "Trans-corporeal Feminisms and the Ethical Space of Nature," *Material Feminisms* 25, no. 2 (2008): 238.
28 Melonçon, "Bringing the Body Back through Performative Phenomenology," 100.
29 Ibid., 99.
30 Lydia McDermott, *Liminal Bodies, Reproductive Health, and Feminist Rhetoric: Searching the Negative Spaces in Histories of Rhetoric* (Lanham, MD: Lexington Books, 2016).
31 Ibid., 15.
32 Ibid., 36.
33 Chion, "The Three Listening Modes," 48.
34 Schafer, *The Soundscape*, 274.
35 Michel Foucault, *The Birth of the Clinic: An Archaeology of Medical Perception* (A. M. Sheridan, Trans.) (London, England: Routledge: 1973/2012), 109.
36 Amy Koerber and Lonie McMichael, "Qualitative Sampling Methods: A Primer for Technical Communicators," *Journal of Business and Technical Communication* 22, no. 4 (2008): 454–73.
37 Joshua Gunn, "On Recording Performance or Speech, the Cry, and the Anxiety of the Fix," *Liminalities: A Journal of Performance Studies* 7 (2011): 1–30.
38 Sendelbach and Funk, "Alarm Fatigue," 378.
39 Michel Foucault. *Discipline and Punish: The Birth of the Prison* (New York: Vintage, 2012), 160.
40 Ibid., 160.
41 Ibid., 166.
42 Schafer, *The Soundscape,* 274.
43 Ibid., 274.
44 Kristin Marie Bivens, Lora Arduser, Candice A. Welhausen, and Michael J. Faris, "A Multisensory Literacy Approach to Biomedical Healthcare Technologies: Aural, Tactile, and Visual Layered Health Literacies," *Kairos* 22, no. 2 (2018). Retrieved from http://kairos.technorhetoric.net/22.2/topoi/bivens-et-al/index.html
45 Debra Hawhee, *Rhetoric in Tooth and Claw: Animals, Language, Sensation* (Chicago, IL: University of Chicago Press, 2017), 54.
46 Chion, "The Three Listening Modes," 49.
47 Linden Gledhill, Cymatics, standing sound waves. Photograph. 2016. Used with permission. https://www.flickr.com/photos/13084997@N03/24654244819/in/album-72157664382425281/
48 Bivens, Arduser, Welhausen, and Faris, "A Multisensory Literacy Approach to Biomedical Healthcare Technologies," n.p.
49 @BeautifulNursing, 2022, "NCLEX TIP: HIGH ALERT MEDS #fyp #foryou #nurse #nursingstudent #nursingschool #nclex #nclextips #MadewithKAContest #PerfectPrideMovement #xyzbca #medtok #medmonday #nclexprep #nursinghacks #nclexhacks." TikTok, June 7, 2022. https://www.tiktok.com/@beautifulnursing/video/7106281561514954030
50 Bivens, Arduser, Welhausen, and Faris, "A Multisensory Literacy Approach to Biomedical Healthcare Technologies," n.p.
51 Ibid.
52 @nursesushi, 2021, "Alarm fatigue is high these days #icu #icurn #criticalcare #rn #nurse #covid #covid19 #vaccinessavelives." TikTok, August 19, 2021. https://www.tiktok.com/@nurse_sushi/video/6998078138420890886
53 Sendelbach and Funk, "Alarm Fatigue."
54 Camellia Torabizadeh, Amirhossein Yousefinya, Farid Zand, Mahnaz Rakhshan, and Mohammad Fararooei, "A Nurses' Alarm Fatigue Questionnaire: Development and Psychometric Properties," *Journal of Clinical Monitoring and Computing* 31, no. 6 (2017): 1305–12.

55 Katarzyna Lewandowska, Magdalena Weisbrot, Aleksandra Cieloszyk, Wioletta Mędrzycka-Dąbrowska, Sabina Krupa, and Dorota Ozga, "Impact of Alarm Fatigue on the Work of Nurses in an Intensive Care Environment—A Systematic Review," *International Journal of Environmental Research and Public Health* 17, no. 22 (2020): 8409.

56 Torabizadeh, Yousefinya, Zand, Rakhshan, and Fararooei, "A Nurses' Alarm Fatigue Questionnaire."

57 Keith J. Ruskin, and Dirk Hueske-Kraus, "Alarm Fatigue: Impacts On Patient Safety," *Current Opinion in Anesthesiology* 28, no. 6 (2015): 685–90.

58 Emalie M. Petersen and Cindy L. Costanzo, "Assessment of Clinical Alarms Influencing Nurses' Perceptions of Alarm Fatigue," *Dimensions of Critical Care Nursing* 36, no. 1 (2017): 36–44.

59 Torabizadeh, Yousefinya, Zand, Rakhshan, and Fararooei, "A Nurses' Alarm Fatigue Questionnaire."

60 Ok Min Cho, Hwasoon Kim, Young Whee Lee, and Insook Cho, "Clinical Alarms in Intensive Care Units: Perceived Obstacles of Alarm Management and Alarm Fatigue in Nurses," *Healthcare Informatics Research* 22, no. 1 (2016): 46–53.

61 @nursesushi, 2021, "Alarm fatigue is high these days #icu #icurn #criticalcare #rn #nurse #covid #covid19 #vaccinessavelives."

62 Lewandowska, Weisbrot, Cieloszyk, Mędrzycka-Dąbrowska, Krupa, and Ozga, "Impact of Alarm Fatigue on the Work of Nurses in an Intensive Care Environment," 8409.

63 Jones, "Alarm Fatigue a Top Patient Safety Hazard," 178.

64 Wallis, "Alarm Fatigue Linked to Patient's Death," 16.

65 Jones, "Alarm Fatigue a Top Patient Safety Hazard," para. 3.

66 Ibid., para. 4.

67 Bradford D. Winters, Maria M. Cvach, Christopher. P. Bonafide, Xiao. Hu, Avinash Konkani, Michael. F. O'Connor ... and Sandra L. Kane-Gill, "Technological Distractions (Part 2): A Summary of Approaches to Manage Clinical Alarms with Intent to Reduce Alarm Fatigue," *Critical Care Medicine* 46, no. 1 (2018): 130–7.

68 Ibid., 133.

69 Cooren, "The Selection of Agency as a Rhetorical Device," 23.

70 Anne Frances Wysocki, "Unfitting Beauties of Transducing Bodies," in *Rhetorics and Technologies: New Directions in Writing and Communication*, ed. Stuart A. Selber (Columbia, SC: University of South Carolina Press, 2010), 104.

71 Chion, Michel, "The Three Listening Modes," *The Sound Studies Reader*, ed. Jonathan Sterne (New York: Routledge, 2012), 48–53.

72 Rice, "Learning to Listen."

73 Harris and Van Drie, "Sharing Sound," 98.

74 Foucault, 150, *Discipline and Punish*, 160.

75 Anne Frances Wysocki, "Introduction: Into Between—in Composition in Mediation," in *Composing Media Composing Embodiment*, eds. Kristin L. Arola and Anne Francis Wysocki (Boulder, CO: University Press of Colorado, 2012), 3.

5 Behaving as Responsible Researchers in Sonic Health, Healing, and Hospital Spaces

Scott and Melonçon describe one of many questions of concern for scholars in RHM: How do we engage health and medical practices and their stakeholders, ethically and responsively?[1] In this chapter, I offer two intertwined responses involving behaving ethically and responsively *toward* health and medical stakeholders—nurses, parents, and other caregivers in NICU—and behaving ethically and responsively in health, healing, and hospital contexts *as* researchers. Since non-discursive, material, influential elements, such as sound, shape action intentionally and unintentionally, responses to Scott and Melonçon's question require accepting my proposition that hearing and feeling bodies in health, healing, and hospital contexts are accountable for what they hear—and can be—by acting as earwitnesses.[2] Earwitnessing is a mark of responsible, ethical researcher behavior that contributes to understanding the rhetoric of the "… passively material"[3] by "prioritizing the bodily experiences of both researchers and participants"[4] and "consider[ing] [the researcher's] … responsibility to the people and communities represented by … [rhetorical] research."[5]

The question driving the chapter arises from a research concept and practice I call sound in all research (SiAR): how can researchers who engage in fieldwork—or individuals who work with those who do—behave responsibly toward sound (or its absence) and its likely effects in research spaces? I provide a rationale for attending to sonic dimensions in fieldwork and research while also acknowledging rhetorical instantiations of the sensorium as complete or whole regarding available senses, which vary from person to person. I offer rhetorically infused, sonic fieldwork practices to integrate alongside other common qualitative data collection methods, such as observation and interview, and a constellation of research practices for acting as earwitnesses while ear-ring[6]—a pedagogical practice that "involves focusing on a particular kind of audible information"[7]—when possible while engaging in fieldwork. The aim is for those with and without acoustic expertise to integrate collecting, analyzing, and attending to sound (and silence or absence of sound) into fieldwork. I also present a heuristic based on SiAR for those who are clinicians in the field—nurses and respiratory therapists among others.

DOI: 10.4324/9781032724416-5

According to Schafer, "the soundscape researcher is concerned with changes in perception and behavior."[8] Along with a constellation of research practices for acting as earwitnesses I offer, I provide heuristic statements and questions for prompting practitioners to consider how hearing, feeling bodies in health, healing, and hospital contexts can optimally engage sound from healthcare technologies and within health and healing soundscapes—a commitment as a rhetorical researcher emanating from sonic phenomena I encountered during my own fieldwork. By considering the source of sound and its impact in fieldwork in health, healing, and hospital contexts, we can further dimensionalize and sensorially enrich our data collection, research analyses, findings, and implications and—importantly—ethically and responsively attend to what we hear. By resisting an ableist ocular centrism,[9] acknowledging sound in our research, and reconfiguring vantage points to incorporate sonic dimensions, we can address a sensory hegemony and sound as discipline for bodies. Just as we are responsible for what we see when we conduct fieldwork, we are also responsible for what we hear beyond spoken statements. Ultimately, sound and rhetoric work together to represent and understand action and sensory information during fieldwork more deeply.

The following questions help illuminate and operationalize the integrated medico-sonic theorization mediated by rhetoric that I offer through SiAR:

- How does sound discipline bodies in hospital contexts?
- What value does attending to sound in health and healing offer and to whom?
- How can ocular centrism or visualism be decentered?
- What are researcher obligations related to sound?
- How can researchers conducting fieldwork in hospital contexts act as earwitnesses?

Sound as Discipline in Hospital Contexts

Sound disciplines all bodies in conventional, science-based, allopathic Western health system hospitals and other related contexts. Foucault defines *discipline* as a consistent control over bodies, their movements, their actions, and even whole populations.[10] In an interview translated from French to English by Leonard Mayhew between Roger-Pol Droit and Foucault that appeared in the Parisian newspaper *Le Monde* in 1975, Foucault described prison as

a rigorous regulation of space, because the guard can and must see everything. It is also the rigid regulation of the use of time hour by hour. Finally, it involves regulation of the slightest bodily movements or change of position.[11]

During the interview, Foucault explained the role of surveillance in prisons, as "the control and identification of individuals, the regulation of their movements, activity, and effectiveness."[12] Foucault also asked—and quite importantly for my argument here about sound as discipline—"What is so astonishing ... about the fact that our prisons resemble our factories, schools, military bases, and hospitals—all of which in turn resemble prisons?"[13] In the interview, which draws from Foucault's groundbreaking historical philosophical work in *Discipline and Punish,*[14] Foucault explains how discipline in prisons provides "day-by-day power over bodies"[15] as "a subtle coercion"[16] and "an infinitesimal power over the active body"[17] for "docility-utility"[18]—a phenomenon similar to how sound can function in hospital contexts.

As auditory environments within conventional hospitals, sounds work rhetorically to reinforce science-based, allopathic, Western health—the predominant medical system that treats symptoms and diseases with drugs, interventions, and operations—understandings of the body. Conventional Western medicine frames or disciplines bodies and their real and rhetorical movements and activities in such rhetorical ecologies. For example, medical devices that dispense medications require vocal sounds for use. The "can you witness?" question asked from RN to RN demonstrates *rhetorical ventriloquism*—"the various ways ... human interactants make certain entities (collectives, procedures, policies, ideologies, etc.) speak in their name and vice versa."[19] The "can you witness?" question represents a nursing procedure based on a hospital policy. Sound disciplines bodies by controlling their actions: the actions of the RNs, as well as the actions or reactions from hospitalized bodies—the infants.

Alaimo's material feminist concept *trans-corporeality*—"the time-space where human corporeality, in all its material fleshiness, is inseparable from 'nature' or 'environment'"[20]—demonstrates and succinctly captures how bodies can be freed from such discipline since bodies are not separate from their environments and the body's sensory experiences are formed by and contribute to the environment. When sound disciplines bodies in hospital contexts, those bodies respond by action, inaction, or reaction. For example, a hospitalized infant's sneeze.[21] In my fieldwork in a NICU in the southwestern United States, I reported:

One day as I waited, a baby—a grower—who was surveilled with a physiological monitor was sleeping in an open crib and sneezed. Her physiological monitor alarmed. As the monitor alarmed, she stirred and briefly woke.

[...]. The baby's alarm was not attended to because almost as fast as it sounded, it stopped—it created distracting alarm noise for an unimportant clinical event, not purposeful alarm sound for an important clinical event.[22]

Hospitalized infants easily become Foucault's docile bodies in hospital contexts because they are inherently vulnerable. Their bodies are watched through the medical gaze,[23] which separates the body into its parts, functions, and conditions, and disciplined by devices and tools, such as physiological monitors that surveil the infant's body, derive power from the medical gaze, and make sounds and noises with rhetorical power emanating from conventional science-based, allopathic Western medical systems. The medical gaze is accompanied by a rhetorically ventriloquized medical voice also capable of disciplining docile bodies. In most cases, especially outside hospital contexts, infant sneezes do not wake the slumbering. Yet, the "day-by-day power"[24] sound demonstrates "over bodies"[25] rhetorically works as "a subtle coercion"[26] to control and regulate body movements in hospital contexts. Since the body was surveilled by a physiological monitor, when the infant sneezed, the monitor's synchretic interpretation of the sneeze—the visual display of the sneeze and its impact on the body's vital functions heard through the beep-beep-beeps the monitor emits—woke the body it surveilled. Although it is certain that healthcare technologies and medical devices that emit sound help the bodies they inspect, it is also certain they disrupt and can harm those same bodies. In this case, it disrupted the sleeping infant.

As another example, medical devices, such as alarming intravenous (IV) pumps, caused bodily movement and action for new parents in a NICU. Recall that "after [audibly] complaining about the [IV] alarm to the mother, the father moved quickly to go find a nurse, causing him to trip and fall on the ground (as I witnessed through the gap between the curtain and floor)."[27] In this instance, the sound from the medical device disciplined the father by prompting his action and reaction to the IV pump's alarm. The medical device or IV pump's alarm sound demonstrated the "subtle coercion"[28] and "infinitesimal power over the active body"[29] for "docility-utility"[30]—the father's active body was disciplined by subtle coercion from infinitesimal power from the alarm sound. The NICU context disciplines physicians, nurses, respiratory therapists, parents, infants; it disciplines bodies—docile bodies—receptive to the power contained within the hospital context.

Listening as Rhetorical Shorthand for Attention

By attending to sound in fieldwork or SiAR, scholars expose and displace ocular centrism and invite attention to other available senses, possibly freeing the body from conventional science-based, allopathic Western healthcare's discipline by sound (and sight). For example, exposing and addressing sound in research sites "helps counter ocular centric (modeled on vision as dominant sensory modality) conceptions"[31]—an argument Steve Goodman makes about accounting for vibrational ecologies in cyberspace. More simply in the words of naturalist and birder Michael O'Brien, "Our eyes can only see what's in front of us, more or less, but we can hear sounds from every direction,"[32] depending on an individual's available senses. As an example, take ornithology or the study of birds. Ocular centrism examines only the visual aesthetic of the bird; yet sidelining or omitting the sounds birds make, considers the feel of bird feathers and engages other available senses to provide other sensory experiences. When we prioritize one available sense, we can obscure others. For instance, rhetorically considering birds further enhances how we sensorially engage cooked turkeys on the dining room tables of meat-eating families in the United States (or around the world) on Thanksgiving Thursday or the promise of songs to remove us from our roosts by *gökotta*—birdsongs on pre-dawn mornings in Sweden. In these ways, birds are experienced by other available senses, such as tasting or hearing, which can deprioritize ocular centrism or visualism and resist sensory hegemony or the domination of one sense.

As Kessler wrote, "We must rhetorically and reflectively listen if we want to ethically engage with each other's lived experiences, particularly in the contexts of health and medicine,"[33] while also encouraging "theories and approaches [...] to focus on the perspectives, perceptions, interpretations, even descriptions of a singular, stable reality."[34] As the previous chapters demonstrate, "listening" is a stand in for such attention; a rhetorical shorthand for giving attention or drawing attention to what counts, what is worthy of noting or amplifying. Decentering visualism or ocular centrism in fieldwork also makes room for what the authors of "Deaf Qualitative Health Research: Leveraging Technology to Conduct Linguistically and Sociopolitcally Appropriate Methods of Inquiry" argue: a paradigm shift from capturing just spoken language to using visual language in health research,[35] which more fully, ethically, and responsively engages with people and their available sensoriums. They suggest six steps to reform qualitative methods for including deaf and deafness into health research from forming the research team to collecting and uploading data into qualitative analysis software to analyzing and disseminating results to deaf and scientific communities.[36] I suggest that an SiAR approach can account for sound's presence or absence and hearing bodies and deafness.

Yet, non-discursive sensory elements, such as smell and sound, are captured and analyzed differently than discursive text- or language-based discourse, such as American Sign Language (ASL). In ancient health and healing systems, rhetoric preserved sound in text through rhetorical devices, such as simile and metaphor, in a similar state that froze olfactory elements in visual miasmatic disease etiologies.[37] In both instances, a stable reality to interpret from is impractical and impossible; however, we can interpret senses through more stable visual and textual—synchretic—means, "even [if] one's own 'individual' experience and understanding of one's body is mediated by science, medicine, epidemiology, and the swirl of subcultures, organizations, Web sites, and magazines ..."[38] The integration of the sonic with rhetoric provides such an opportunity, such a textual record to draw from. The introduction to *Field Rhetoric* argues for "immersing oneself in the dynamic living, breathing ecologies that give rise to rhetoric and its work," adding it "enhances the capacity to understand and observe rhetoric as a three-dimensional, situated force"[39]; I agree and extend rhetoric's role to the sonic in fieldwork where rhetoric enriches "the material turn" and the possibilities from "look[ing] beyond the human body" "to understand the fullest most inventive capacities of rhetoric."[40] In *Field Work*, they offer their collection of field methodologies, ontologies, and interventions as "engaging in and with the places of persuasion for understanding utterances in context, understanding objects of study in situ, and offering opportunities for engagement and intervention" with rhetoric as the frame.[41] Conceptually and practically, SiAR provides fieldworkers opportunities for engaging in and understanding research site capacity related to soundscapes, sound, and silence.

Sound in All Research

Ultimately, how can researchers who conduct fieldwork account for sonicity? SiAR is an approach that integrates sound, silence, and listening into all fieldwork—from planning and engaging with participants through publication and presentation; it involves planning, conducting, analyzing, and reporting research. I share recommendations for incorporating SiAR into each of these stages of research.

To advocate for researchers and scholars and hospital administrators, clinicians, and health and patient advocates alike to act as earwitnesses—an embodied practice and sensorial act to focus attention on sound and perhaps other available senses—in research contexts, SiAR offers a collection of sound and sense-oriented preparation, fieldwork practices, analytical processes, and habits and behaviors for reporting and considering sound. Listening or attention to sonic elements presents rhetoric as a field researcher's practical tool—one "of perception and orientation"[42] when paired with intentional attention to sonicity from rhetorical and feminist materialist perspectives. By accounting for our bodies and the sensoria's available senses, rhetoric transforms from textually presented, culturally derived metaphors and similes to empirically recorded information noted during fieldwork. For example, rhetoric transforms words into sound when Majno replicated a metaphor of lung sounds "as ... boiling inside like vinegar,"[43] he noted that boiling vinegar sounded like "rushing, crackling noise, quite unlike that of boiling water and comparing very well with the sound heard over a lung when fluid obstructs the finest bronchi."[44] Rhetoric allowed Majno and myself—and other hearing humans—to reach through time and reproduce a lung sound described centuries ago. With assistance from rhetorical devices, such as simile, we can replicate sounds and understand how they have been shaped across a vast expanse of time. With rhetoric, it is also possible to share our sonic understandings and perceptions of sound in health, healing, and hospital contexts within various discourse communities. SiAR is designed to assist fieldworkers do just that.

Planning: Research Protocols and Casing the Scene

In most cases, when research is conducted among humans, ethical reviews of research are required. During the review, research plans are assessed for respect of persons, beneficence, and justice—three key ethical principles. Next, I provide several suggestions for incorporating SiAR in research protocols, as well as preparing for fieldwork by casing the scene.

Research Protocols

From the perspective of SiAR and to show respect for persons and demonstrate justice, *provide accessible recruitment and consent materials, curate a sign-only language interview environment for deaf participants,* and *prepare participants for digital recordings.*

Provide accessible recruitment and consent materials. If you use a video to recruit participants in your study, use closed captioning and voiceover to accompany any audio in the video. Provide digital and physical consent materials as early as possible. Employ a certified deaf interpreter[45] to assist during the consent process.

Curate a sign-only language interview environment for deaf participants. Since deaf people may participate in your study, include language in your study protocol, such as "Since 'whenever possible a sign-only environment is favored'[46] by deaf people, interviews will be video recorded and conducted in [sign language]."

Prepare participants for digital recordings. If you intend to digitally capture elements of the soundscape—the "acoustic [or sonic] environment[s],"[47]— include such information in your protocol and written consent materials. For example, "to best describe the context or scene from the research site, I will digitally record sounds from the acoustic environment. I will tell you when I turn on and off the digital recorder; you can ask me turn off the recording at any time for any reason."

Casing the Scene

When planning fieldwork and working with human participants, *casing the scene* and *modifying or manipulating our visual and aural experiences* while doing so can make unfamiliar research contexts familiar and provide a sense what is going on[48] prior to officially beginning fieldwork.

Casing the scene helps researchers study for acting decorously[49] or preparing for the "test of acculturation"[50] so, we can "give meaning to the actors and actions"[51] in restricted areas, such as hospital units, where we conduct fieldwork. By casing the scene, I also suggest we can tune into different aspects of our research sites prior to conducting fieldwork and make ourselves familiar with and within those sites.

Only with permission from gatekeepers or sponsors,[52] I suggest casing the scene—or scouting—prior to engaging in fieldwork[53] in restricted areas, especially while waiting for human research ethics board review and determination. For example, for a microstudy I conducted in a methodology course during my graduate studies, I first cased the scene after sponsors approved my presence—a NICU in the Midwest part of the United States. When I was there, I could ascertain general qualities of the research site: the temperature (in case I needed a sweater), what vantage points might be ideal for observation (so I would be prepared when nearby), the location of the bathroom (for instances when I might need it), and quiet locations with privacy and space for interviews (so I could provide ideal interview conditions for participants).

Modifying our visual and aural experiences when casing the scene so we can prioritize different senses by manipulating our available ones.

When casing the scene, I recommend intentionally modifying your sensory experience by wearing ear plugs and limiting the visual when available and safe to do so. Once I received written permission from gatekeepers—the NICU supervisor and assistant supervisor—for my microstudy, I was escorted to an unoccupied nursery. I wore earplugs—the closest item for acting like earlids—so I could not hear conversations (or healthcare technologies), and I focused on what I saw. Then I removed the earplugs and closed my eyes to focus on what I heard. Since I sought to observe communicative exchanges between nurses and parents of infants hospitalized in NICUs, I focused on active areas where these exchanges occurred and recorded them with an X in a crude drawing of the NICU in my fieldnotes. If permissible by gatekeepers or sponsors, you might consider taking photos, as well.

Conducting: Interviews and Observations

By casing the scene, ideal interview and observation vantage points are likely known, which supports integrating SiAR elements from research protocols, such as securing optimal interview spaces, in fieldwork. For interviews and observations during fieldwork, I offer three question sets to better understand the soundscape and sensory experiences of participants. By thinking through and responding to questions such as these, more sonic and sensory information can help dimensionalize field research sites and research reports from them.

Interviewing Participants

The first question set aims to provide both ideal sonic experiences for hearing participants and sufficient and preferred methods for communicating with deaf participants.

Hearing participants. Generally, when conducting interviews with hearing participants and applying SiAR, it means controlling for potential sonic shrapnel that might interfere with the interview and sensitizing interview locations for participant comfort. Consider the following questions when preparing to interview hearing participants.

- Have I provided a quiet location for paying attention[54] and easy listening and speaking during interviews with participants?
- Have I provided audio and/or text-based printed or digital interview schedule or guide[55] for participants in advance?
- Have I provided a method for participants to audio record interviews or write down their thoughts during interviews for their own comfort?
- Have I looked for and acted upon signs of engagement and disengagement, such as microwithdrawals of consent,[56] during interviews with participants?

Deaf participants. Obtain active involvement or advice from deaf community advisors,[57] if possible, especially if you intend to recruit deaf participants. Prior to conducting research with deaf participants, I recommend carefully reading Anderson and colleague's exceptional article "Deaf Qualitative Health Research: Leveraging Technology and Sociopolitcally Appropriate Methods of Inquiry," as well as seeking answers to the following questions and preparing ideal conditions for interviews with deaf participants.

- Have I provided a certified deaf interpreter for deaf participants?[58]
- Have I provided audio and/or text-based printed or digital interview schedule or guide[59] for participants in advance?
- Have I provided a sign-only environment and limited the number of hearing people during interviews with deaf participants?[60]
- With participant permission, have I video and audio recorded multiple streams of the interviews?[61]
- Have I looked for and acted upon signs of engagement and disengagement, such as microwithdrawals of consent, during interviews with participants?

Observing Participants

The second question set promotes Chion's three modes of listening—causal, reduced, and semantic[62] with the aim to characterize the soundscape, including keynote sounds, signals, and soundmarks, by acting as earwitnesses.

- What sounds and noises comprise the soundscape?
- When is the soundscape silent?
- How do participants experience the soundscape, sounds, and silence?

- What are the soundscape's keynote sounds; signals; and soundmarks?
- What do causal, reduced, and semantic listening help understand?

When listening in causal, reduced, and semantic modes, field researchers can *earwitness* by testifying to what they hear[63] and—as I suggest—act as sonically responsible researchers. Recall *causal listening* determines sources of sounds, *reduced listening* characterizes sounds, and *semantic listening* interprets sound's messages.[64] *Keynote sounds* are "those heard … continuously or frequently" and even unconsciously[65]; a *soundscape*"[66] is the sonic environment and *signals* are "any sound to which attention is particularly directed"[67]; *soundmarks* are "a community sound which is unique or possesses qualities which make it specially regarded or noticed by the people in that community."[68] Keynote sounds are taken for granted and comparable to noise or unintentional, possibly disruptive sound, while soundmarks are more likely to be sonically noticed, intentional, purposeful sound.

Sonic records are essential for SiAR and involve digital audio and textual recordings of sounds to provide context and support for sonic impressions. When observing and acting as an earwitness during fieldwork, record your EARWITNESS FIELDNOTES—the keynote, signals and soundmarks that populate a field site's soundscape tracked along with causal, reduced, and semantic modes of listening. For later confirmation during interviews or when member checking or validating[69] findings during analysis, record your *sonic impression* and ask your research participants about them. Within SiAR fieldnotes or EARWITNESS FIELDNOTES, reserve space to systematically collect information about the field site's soundscape, such as the example in Table 5.1.

In EARWITNESS FIELDNOTES, record day and time and listening mode, noting that in certain field sites semantic listening requires checking with experts for meaning, while causal and reduced can be likely ascertained during fieldwork. However, as fieldworkers become more familiar with field sites,

Table 5.1 Example earwitness fieldnote entry applying SiAR in a hospital context.

EARWITNESS FIELDNOTES
causal = source of sound; *reduced* = characteristics of sound; *semantic* = message of sound
keynote sound = continuous; frequent; *signal* = needs attention; *soundmark* = unique community sound

	LISTENING MODE	CAUSAL	REDUCED	SEMANTIC	SONIC IMPRESSION
date & time	sound type				
05/12/2024 9:12 am	☑ keynote sound ☑ signal ☐ soundmark	ventilator	Louder and louder ding, ding, ding. >30 seconds	??	Sound seems ignored, yet sometimes noticed.

Soundnotes: Digital recording of sound in folder 3. If parent and nurse participants agree to interviews, ask about sound and what it meant.

it is possible they will see trends across EARWITNESS FIELDNOTES and benefit from clarifications from interview participants. For determining sources of sound from causal listening, I recommend using an existing classification system from either Schafer or R. Bruce Lindsay[70,71]; Schafer's system includes broader categories, such as natural, human, sounds and society, mechanical, quiet and silence, and sounds as indicators.[72] As an example, Schafer categorizes human sounds into voice, body, and clothing; human voice sounds are further subdivided into speaking, calling, whispering, crying, screaming, among others.[73] Since SiAR offers opportunities for fieldworkers with some acoustic knowledge or expertise to incorporate sound (and silence) into collecting, analyzing, and attending to sound in research, Schafer provides six qualities of settings that can assist describing characteristics of sound for reduced listening mode: distance from sound, intensity of sound in decibels, whether the sound was distinct and to what degree, ambiance, frequency of sound, and environmental factors, such as reverberation presence and length and echo.[74]

The Lindsay's 1963 wheel of acoustics[75] is physics-based. Four larger categories make up Lindsay's "The Science of Acoustics" wheel: earth sciences, engineering, life sciences, and arts. Medicine, physiology, and psychology comprise life sciences and communication is categorized under speech and music in a larger arts category. Lindsay's wheel of acoustics is another tool for causal listening—a tool to assist fieldworkers when recording EARWITNESS FIELDNOTES. Although the categories are broader and more encompassing than Schafer's categorizations, using Lindsay's wheel of acoustics can possibly show connections and overlap among various acoustical components, as well as disciplinary boundaries. However, for those without acoustic expertise or ready use of acoustical terminology, I suggest using rhetorical onomatopoeia to create textual records and descriptions of sounds for reduced listening, which is a good starting place rooted in the evolution of medico-sonic knowledge I theorize.

There is also a possibility of overlap regarding sound types. For example, depending on the listener and mode of listening, a ventilator—like the example from the previous chapter—could be a keynote sound, signal, *and* soundmark. In hospital contexts—or other field sites—when permissible, make digital audio recordings for later analysis; then produce written transcripts of alarming physiological monitors described with onomatopoeia, such as "Louder ding, ding, ding/... Ping-ding, ping-ding, ping-ding, ping-ding from a monitor/... Ding ding ding ding ding ding ding (fast-paced)" of a healthcare monitor.[76] The written description can be initially handwritten onomatopoeically in EARWITNESS FIELDNOTES, and subsequently checked against digital audio recordings later.

If you have an iPhone, consider downloading the accurate,[77] award-winning, free National Institute for Occupational Safety and Health (NIOSH) Sound Level Meter. The Sound Level Meter includes "professional sound level meters and noise dosimeters"[78] with an accuracy of ±2 decibels A (dBa), which provides a level of loudness for human ears. The Sound Level Meter also comes with a user manual.[79] As field researchers become more familiar with field sites during fieldwork, it is likely they will see trends across EARWITNESS FIELDNOTES and benefit from member checking and clarifications courtesy of interview participants.

Analyzing: Participant Interviews, Digital Recordings, EARWITNESS FIELDNOTES, *and Theoretical Memoing*

After collecting data from interview participants and observations while applying SiAR fieldwork practices, analyzing data includes triangulating sonic findings from participant interviews, digital recordings, and EARWITNESS FIELDNOTES. Yet, prior to starting analysis and after a predetermined segment, such as several hours or one day, I recommend a borrowed and slightly adjusted practice from Kathy Charmaz's grounded theory: theoretical memoing.[80] However, before theoretical memoing, I suggest working with other sources of sound data, such as participant interviews, digital recordings, and EARWITNESS FIELDNOTES.

Participant Interviews

Although research questions and chosen theoretical frameworks are the primary lens used for analyzing data collected during fieldwork, I offer SiAR-oriented analytical processes to account for sound and silence in field sites: *transcribe interviews personally* and *involve deaf community advisors*.

Transcribe interviews personally. In my own research, I found transcription an invaluable process for accounting for sound and soundscapes. There are many opportunities to use artificial intelligence and natural language processing, such as Sonix, otter.ai, or Speak AI, for transcribing digital audio recordings into text; however, I recommend personally transcribing interview digital audio recordings. If doing so is burdensome, I suggest using software like Audiate.

Involve deaf community advisors. If fieldworkers do not know sign language, for interviews with deaf participants the multiple streams of video capturing sign-only interviews require certified deaf interpreters for transcription. When deaf community advisors are involved, they can provide guidance about understanding deaf community and "commonplace experiences" perhaps "taken for granted during the data analysis process."[81]

Digital Recordings

With human research ethical approval, as well as approval from participants, gatekeepers, and research sponsors, digital audio recordings of interviews and observations capture sounds (and silence) of soundscapes for later analysis. However, when sounds become familiar, such as keynote sounds, it can be difficult to notice them during moments of fieldwork.

I recommend fieldworkers *create waveforms of soundscapes* and *characterize sounds with rhetorical devices.*

Create waveforms of soundscapes. Waveforms reveal the shape of sound. If you used sound level meters and noise dosimeters, such as the NIOSH Sound Level Meter app, sound readings from these devices or apps can identify possible sounds and noises worthy of further investigation. I also recommend using a media player, such as Audacity, to import digital audio recordings from observations and interviews, which automatically produce a waveform. After creating waveforms, I suggest a three-part process involving manipulating your senses. If available for modifying, I suggest closing your eyes and listening, putting in earplugs and watching, and viewing and listening simultaneously, depending on available senses.

Characterize sounds with rhetorical devices. Once you have identified important sonic features from soundscapes, such as keynote sounds, signals, and soundmarks, use onomatopoeia, simile, and metaphor to rhetorically describe those sounds. By doing so, these descriptions can be used in transcripts that accompany digital audio recordings, such as mp3 or WAV files, and make sound recordings accessible for blind and deaf people. Transcripts that accompany sound files can also be paired with extended or regular audio descriptions.[82]

EARWITNESS FIELDNOTES

The practice of recording fieldnotes "create the foundation on which our analytical claims are subsequently built."[83] They document[84] and emphasize the "importance of fieldnotes for studies using participant observations."[85] The EARWITNESS FIELDNOTES are integral for applying SiAR conceptually and practically, as well as recording your sonic impressions, which can be member checked or validated and later integrated into your reports of fieldwork, such as presentations, publications, or circulated among the communities involved or engaged with fieldwork.

To make the most of the documentation from EARWITNESS FIELDNOTES, I recommend *sound tracing* and *theoretical memoing.*

Sound tracing. As a unique SiAR analytic process, sound tracing takes the soundscape's keynote sounds, signals, and soundmarks identified in EARWITNESS FIELDNOTES and assumes—one at a time—that each is the impetus for action, speech, or feeling. In tandem with complete field notes and digital audio recordings, sound tracing roughly sketches a sound's rhetorical influence and power.

Once several keynote sounds, signals, and soundmarks are traced, hypothesize how those sounds influenced an action or inaction and perhaps other sensory information participants relied upon to make decisions. Since prioritizing the bodily experiences of both researchers and participants are integral to sensory accounts during fieldwork, consider the following questions when sound tracing:

- How did the soundscape and its sound or silence impact you?
- What other senses, such as olfactory or haptic, contributed to your experience during fieldwork?
- Did you experience affect—"a visceral bodily sensation that is physiological but social"?[86]
- What participants were influenced by specific sounds from the soundscape?
- How are those influential sounds characterized?
- Did participants experience affect?

I recommend sound tracing prior to theoretical memoing and incorporating synthesized conceptualizations from your sound tracing in theoretical memos.

Theoretical memoing. Rhetoric is a powerful tool; it "can offer fieldworkers a keen attunement, for instance, to the notion that ethnographic and field-based accounts of the world are implicitly representational, both analogic and heuristical, and tend to offer situated, multiple truths that circulate within a place."[87] To extend the statement and show its bearing on the sound in research, SiAR formed from rhetorical understandings of the role of sound in health in healing; thus the attunement is actual, as well as analogic and heuristic.

To draw out sound and its possible implications from fieldwork, I recommend theoretical memoing. To start, after a predetermined duration of time in the field, write, draw, or record SiAR-oriented theoretical memos. The memos are meant to generate your thinking related to sound over time during and after fieldwork. As you complete a segment of your research, record your impressions in writing, sketch a drawing, save as a voice note on a digital recording device, or by any method you find useful and appropriate.

Consider the following to extract sonic-related information from your fieldwork.

- Review the segment's EARWITNESS FIELDNOTES for trends or notable outliers worthy of further investigation during the next fieldwork segment, observation, or interview.
- Listen to any digital audio recordings of the soundscape by enacting the three modes of listening: causal, reduced, and semantic.
- Import digital audio recordings into a media player, such as Audacity, to see the sound as waveforms; record what you see in the waveforms, including patterns and silence.
- Endeavor for semantic listening understandings of what you hear.
- Categorize your sonic impressions as adding texture to research questions or not.

- Note any lingering concerns related to the soundscape, silence, keynote sound, signal, or soundmark.
- Determine how research participants might take sound and silence for granted.
- Compare sound and silence across time during fieldwork segments.
- Hypothesize consequences of sound and silence.
- Categorize sounds using either Schafer or Lindsay.

Reporting: Presentations, Publications, Communities, and Social Media

Traditionally, findings from fieldwork are reported during *presentations* or in *publications*, as well as circulated among involved and engaged *communities* and their members. For all kinds of reporting, if possible, when incorporating fieldwork soundscapes into presentations and publications or sharing with involved and engaged communities, consider including audio sound files and waveforms that visually depict and show the shape of sound, or sound's materiality. Both sound files and wave forms can also add multimodal dimensions to findings reported on *social media*.

As an SiAR principle, ethically use original recordings of sounds and voices only when permissible and with written and verbal consent as required by local laws. To make sound recordings accessible, provide captioning and transcripts.

Presentations. During face-to-face presentations, when sharing quotations from participants or sounds from field sites, use original recordings. For example, use rhetorical devices to describe a soundmark, such as beeping physiological monitor in an intensive care unit, then play the digital audio recording. For virtual presentations, ethically integrate original audio recordings and pre-record presentations and later add closed captioning. Pre-recording is beneficial for closed captioning because accuracy can be ensured.

Publications. When possible, publish in journals with capabilities to hyperlink to multimedia files, such as mp3 sound files. Along with mp3 sound files, include accompanying sound files with transcripts and extended or regular audio descriptions.[88] In the text of the article or other published work, use rhetorical devices, such as onomatopoeia, to describe sounds or make comparisons with rhetorical devices, such as simile and metaphor.

Communities. Ethically circulating findings from fieldwork among the communities engaged and involved in fieldwork is an imperative. Regarding sound and sharing the sounds of a community, obtain guidance from field site sponsors, community members, and gatekeepers before circulating sounds, especially sounds of voices, which might be easily identifiable to members of the community.

Social Media. Once digitally available through social media, for example, sounds can be co-opted, adjusted, remixed, or otherwise modified without permission or consent. I recommend talking through the intended digital footprint—or more accurately, digital echo—of sonic content shared on the Internet or through apps versus the unintended digital footprint of multimedia. However, if mp3 or other sound files are shared to accompany publications or announce a virtual presentation, include captioning—with the rhetorical device onomatopoeia—for non-speech sounds, as well as extended or regular audio descriptions.[89]

"Unnecessary noise, then, is the most cruel absence of care which can be inflicted either on sick or well"[90]

According to the World Health Organization (WHO), "Noise is an underestimated threat that can cause a number of short- and long-term health problems."[91] WHO provides guidelines for sound levels to reduce the incidence of such short- and long-term health problems, such as hearing impairment and sleep disturbance.[92] In the WHO "Guidelines for Community Noise" report, it states, "For a good night's sleep, the equivalent sound level should not exceed 30 dB(A) for continuous background noise, and individual noise events exceeding 45 dB(A) should be avoided."[93] However, in a recent 2020 systematic review and meta-analysis—a synthesis of findings related to sound reduction for infants hospitalized in NICUs—Abdulraoof Almadhoob, Arne Ohlsson, and the Cochrane Neonatal Group reported "The sound levels in NICUs often exceed the maximum acceptable level of 45 decibels (dB), recommended by the American Academy of Pediatrics [AAP]."[94] The AAP's recommendation of 45 dBA is the maximum from WHO's recommendation avoiding "individual noise events exceeding 45 dBA." Although dBA recommendations from WHO and AAP diverge, accounting for the sonic experiences in NICUs and other healthcare spaces is likely best approached with SiAR practices concerned with embodied sonic experiences in health, healing, and hospital contexts.

Recognizing sonic experiences in healthcare contexts provides opportunities for more overt and intentional sensory or sensuous training for nurses, parents, and other caregivers alike. Sensuous training contributes to how nurses integrate causal, reduced, and semantic listening to learn and sonically interpret alarms from physiological monitors. In turn, such training also influences how nurses sensuously train parents and other caregivers in hospital contexts, such as NICUs. Our semantic listening interpretations of sounds and noises are informed by the echoes of our prior aural experiences—akin to how literacy is "haunted"[95] by prior experiences with technologies. Interpretations of sounds in NICUs are directly tied to expertise or sonological competence demonstrated via accurate semantic listening ("sensuous training") and influenced ("haunted") by our prior aural experiences and modes of causal, reduced, and semantic listening. For example, such sensuous training can help listeners or viewers—when information is synchretic—identify and distinguish important clinical sounds and visual notifications from unimportant, distracting noises and notifications. In NICU contexts, such sensuous training could better prepare parents and other legal caregivers for caring for their infants outside of the NICU.

Additionally, sensuous training might include tactile or haptic senses. For instance, instead of sonic healthcare technology alarms, with Bluetooth technologies it might be possible for the alarms to tactilely signal by vibrating through a patch on a nurse, parent, or caregiver's arm. Sounds from medical devices also could be musical. A hospitalized electronic musician—Yoko Sen—described her experience with alarms in a hospital "sonic hellscape"[96] through her expertise as a musician:

> ... a cardiac monitor rang out in a tone close to the musical note of C, clashing with a distant device wailing in a high–pitched F sharp, creating what's called the devil's interval, a dissonance so chilling that medieval churches forbade it.[97]

The International Electrotechnical Commission "publishes guidelines for electronic and technical equipment used by hospitals."[98] For their work, they have created medical device tones or "auditory icons"[99] for six bodily, critical functions, which—with more testing—might possibly replace the existing "audio cues"[100] from "bleating"[101] medical devices. By switching and prioritizing a different sense besides the aural to signify important clinical events or making alarms from medical devices musical, it is possible to provide quieter, less dissonant spaces for all hospitalized infants and people to sleep, as well as nurses, parents, and other legal caregivers to contribute and support health in hospitals. Acknowledging our bodies, our sensuous trainings, and our sensorial experiences within healthcare settings such as NICUs can transform noise from sonic hellscapes or soundscapes and sonic shrapnel into more meaningful—even more harmonious—sounds.

Yet, since bodies are disciplined by sound in hospital contexts, how can physicians, nurses, and other clinicians and carers use SiAR practices to unencumber and reduce sound's discipline on bodies? I offer three question sets to demonstrate how clinicians can expose and address sound.

Reducing Noise for Patients, Clinicians, and Visitors

Sonically oriented questions about patients, clinicians, and visitors might integrate hospital and unit policies related to sound, as well as WHO recommendations for dBa and the use of the iPhone NIOSH app. Generally, if the immediate area is noisy and the noise level cannot be controlled, consider encouraging patients to wear noise cancelling headphones or wearing earplugs or earmuffs to dampen the noise if safe to do so.

The following questions involve the least or simplest actions to minimize sound around patients.

- Can I close doors to patient rooms and around the unit, such as nursing report rooms, call rooms, and break rooms, to reduce sounds from surrounding areas?
- Does the door squeak? If so, consider requesting maintenance.
- Is the heating, ventilation, and air condition system making noises? If so, consider requesting maintenance.
- Am I contributing sound unintentionally? For example, are my shoes squeaking? Or do objects jingle in my pockets when I walk?
- Can alarm ranges on physiological monitors, ventilators, and other medical devices be safely adjusted to reflect parameters suitable for patient conditions?
- Are medical devices making other unnecessary noise that can be fixed with maintenance or replacement?
- Is my personal smartphone switched off or silent?
- Have I asked visitors to switch off or silence their smartphones?
- Are pagers set to silent or vibrate?
- For coordination of care processes, such as change of shift report or moving patients within hospital units, am I contributing sound unintentionally, especially when patients are sleeping?
- Is the volume reasonably low for televisions or personal entertainment devices, such as smartphones or tablets, in patient rooms and common areas for visitors, such as waiting rooms? Is the closed captioning turned on?
- Are rolling carts and trolleys, such as those used by maintenance and cafeteria staff or phlebotomists and respiratory therapists, maintained and checked for jingling or rattling sounds? If there are any noises, can those be fixed with maintenance or replacement?

If it is possible, especially for those who work during common sleeping hours between 8:00 pm and 8:00 am, consider using the NIOSH app to measure dBa or noise levels to identify times and locations when WHO recommendations, hospital policies, and other guidelines provide acceptable dBa indicators for sound. If dBa levels exceed recommendations, simple solutions, such as providing noise cancelling headphones for patients while hospitalized or disposable earplugs or earmuffs, can help reduce the noises heard by patients.

Although hospital and other health and healing contexts are unlikely to be silent, quiet is helpful for resting and sleeping for most people. In fact, silence creates a different problem—one where patients, staff, clinicians, and visitors possibly feel isolated and disconnected. If a hospital or unit or ward has a sound policy or hours reserved for quiet, ensure those policies are known by clinicians, employees, patients, and visitors. Provide quiet hour policies in writing and as a visual, as well as verbal and visual reminders when staff, patients, and visitors arrive at the hospital and unit or ward.

Behaving Ethically and Responsively in Health, Healing, and Hospital Contexts as Researchers

Studying soundscapes and sonic experiences, provides an opportunity to sensorially enrich our knowledge and share sonic information about field research sites. Non-discursive, material yet influential and possibly helpful and harmful elements, such as sound, shape action intentionally and unintentionally; sound in conventional Western health system hospitals and other similar science-based Western contexts discipline bodies within those environments. Since rhetoric and rhetorical understandings help make sense of sound and the body, researchers engaged in fieldwork are responsible for sound and its likely effects in research spaces—just as we are responsible for what we see; we are also responsible for what we hear. Elsewhere I argued for prioritizing the bodily experiences of both researcher and participants. By heeding sound and considering its source and impact in field research contexts, especially in hospitals and other health and healing spaces, we dimensionalize and sensorially enrich our research analyses, findings, and implications. Using SiAR practices helps add such texture to our research and our participant experiences during fieldwork in hospitals.

In their collection *Text + Field: Innovations in Rhetorical Method*, Sara L. McKinnon, Robert Asen, Karma R. Chávez, and Robert Glen Howard list a selection of field methods: interviews, focus groups, observation, personal narrative, ethnography, autoethnography, oral history interviews, performance, thematic analysis, iterative analysis, and grounded theory.[102] They claim when fieldwork is infused by rhetoric or rhetoric is integrated into field work, these merged research practices "[encourage] engagement with audiences" that "may bolster rhetorical understandings of audiences as active participants in processes of meaning making."[103] In health, healing, and hospital contexts, audiences are healthcare clinicians, such as registered nurses, physicians, and respiratory therapists, as well as parents, siblings, legal caregivers, such as foster or adoptive parents, and other support people. I extend McKinnon, Asen, Chávez, Howard and their collection offerings with SiAR— the R could easily be squared (SiAR^2) and stand for sound in all rhetoric research during fieldwork.

Acknowledging sound is also an act of feminist rhetorical research—one that harkens back to a statement from chapter 1: My feminism means drawing attention to what counts, what is worthy of noting or amplifying. As I have endeavored to demonstrate in these pages, sound counts; sound disciplines; sound matters. To be certain, sound in health, healing, and hospital contexts can be intentional and helpful, providing diagnostic, prognostic, and therapeutic possibilities, while noise is unintentional and potentially disruptive, yet also revealing. The rhetorical roots of sound in health and healing relied on onomatopoeia, simile, and metaphor. Over thousands of years, a medico-sonic, rhetorically-mediated lexicon comprised of similes and metaphors provided medical education for using the sounds of bodies to diagnose them, then later treat, make predictions about, and discipline them. When integrated, rhetoric and sound have played a pivotal role in health and healing systems since just prior to time in memorial.

In a chapter from *Sounding Composition*, Ceraso explores sound design and automotive acoustical engineering. She discusses how consumer products are sonically designed for experiences. From the sound of a turn signal to a horn, she argues acoustical sound engineers shape sounds; those sounds "contribute to drivers' feelings about cars"—the driving experience.[104] Ceraso contends automotive acoustical engineers "must consider how sound works with other sensory and material features of the car, as well as how sound affects the bodily experiences of drivers and pedestrians."[105] In addition to alarm fatigue and desensitization to alarms in hospitals, hospital acoustical environments are health and healing concerns and also rhetorical ones. Noise levels in science-based, allopathic Western biomedical hospitals, such as @nurse_sushi's intensive care unit, prioritize the knowing about the body, disciplining the body, yet not the body itself. Either limiting or reducing sound levels or designing acoustic experiences using human-centered approaches[106] is insufficient for "accomodat[ing] the complex multisensory and atmospheric conditions that are central parts of the noise problem in shared hospital spaces."[107] Since our senses exist and make sense in multi-sensory sensoria, rhetorically considering the fuller experiences of all bodies and how bodies are disciplined in hospital contexts relies on attending to each sense separately and together. In response, I offer SiAR or SiAR^2 to begin to systematically account for sound in health and healing fieldwork sites, such as hospitals.

Notes

1 J. Blake Scott and Melonçon, Lisa, "Manifesting Methodologies for the Rhetoric of Health & Medicine," in *Methodologies for the Rhetoric of Health & Medicine*, eds. Lisa Melonçon and J. Blake Scott (New York, NY: Routledge: 2018), 15.
2 R. Murray Schafer, *The Soundscape: Our Sonic Environment and the Tuning of the World* (Rochester, VT: Destiny Books, 1977/1994).
3 Rickert, *Ambient Rhetoric*, 3.
4 Kristin Marie Bivens, "Rhetorically Listening for Microwithdrawals of Consent in Research Practice," in *Methodologies for the Rhetoric of Health & Medicine*, eds. Lisa Melonçon and J. Blake Scott pp. 138–56, (New York: Routledge, 2017), 147.
5 Sara L. McKinnon, Sara L., Robert Asen, Karma R. Chávez, and Robert Glenn Howard, eds. *Text + Field: Innovations in Rhetorical Method* (College Station, PA: Penn State Press, 2016), Kindle edition, n.p.

6 Steph Ceraso, *Sounding Composition: Multimodal Pedagogies for Embodied Listening* (Pittsburgh, PA: University of Pittsburgh Press, 2018), 6.

7 Ibid., 6.

8 Schafer, *The Soundscape*, 89.

9 Graham, S. Scott, "Agency and the Rhetoric of Medicine: Biomedical Brain Scans and the Ontology of Fibromyalgia," *Technical Communication Quarterly* 18, no. 4 (2009): 376–404.

10 Michel Foucault, *Discipline and Punish: The Birth of the Prison* (New York: Vintage, 2012).

11 Roger-Pol Droit, "Michel Foucault, on the Role of Prisons," *The New York Times on the Web*. Leonard Mayhew (transl.). (5 August 1975). Retrieved from https://archive.nytimes.com/www.nytimes.com/books/00/12/17/specials/foucault-prisons.html, para. 7.

12 Droit, "Michel Foucault, on the Role of Prisons," para. 17.

13 Ibid., para. 8.

14 Foucault, *Discipline and Punish*.

15 Droit, "Michel Foucault, on the Role of Prisons," para. 17.

16 Foucault, *Discipline and Punish*, 137.

17 Ibid.

18 Foucault, *Discipline and Punish*, 137.

19 François Cooren, "The Selection of Agency as a Rhetorical Device: Opening up the Scene of Dialogue through Ventriloquism," *Dialogue and Rhetoric* (2008): 23–24.

20 Stacy Alaimo, "Trans-corporeal Feminisms and the Ethical Space of Nature," *Material Feminisms* 25, no. 2 (2008): 238.

21 Bivens, Arduser, Welhausen, and Faris, "A Multisensory Literacy Approach to Biomedical Healthcare Technologies: Aural, Tactile, and Visual Layered Health Literacies," n.p.

22 Ibid.

23 Michel Foucault, *The Birth of the Clinic: An Archaeology of Medical Perception* (A. M. Sheridan, Trans.) (London, England: Routledge: 1973/2012), 109.

24 Droit, "Michel Foucault, on the Role of Prisons," para. 17.

25 Ibid.

26 Foucault, *Discipline and Punish*, 137.

27 Bivens, Arduser, Welhausen, and Faris, "A Multisensory Literacy Approach to Biomedical Healthcare Technologies: Aural, Tactile, and Visual Layered Health Literacies," n.p.

28 Foucault, *Discipline and Punish*, 137.

29 Ibid.

30 Ibid.

31 Goodman, Steve, "The Ontology of Vibrational Force," *The Sound Studies Reader* (2012): 72.

32 Marc Devokaitis, "How to Bird by Ear: Q&A with Michael O'Brien and Louise Zemaitis," *Living Bird*, 15 April, 2015. https://www.allaboutbirds.org/news/how-to-bird-by-ear-qa-with-michael-obrien-and-louise-zemaitis/

33 Kessler, *Stigma Stories*, ix.

34 Ibid., 51.

35 Melissa L. Anderson, Timothy Riker, Kurt Gagne, Stephanie Hakulin, Todd Higgins, Jonah Meehan, Elizabeth Stout, Emma Pici-D'Ottavio, Kelsey Cappetta, and Kelly S. Wolf Craig, "Deaf Qualitative Health Research: Leveraging Technology to Conduct Linguistically and Sociopolitically Appropriate Methods of Inquiry," *Qualitative Health Research* 28, no. 11 (2018): 1813–24.

36 Anderson, Riker, Gagne, Hakulin, Higgins, Meehan, Stout, Pici-D'Ottavio, Cappetta, and Craig, "Deaf Qualitative Health Research," 1817–1822.

37 Emily Winderman, Robert Mejia, and Brandon Rogers, "All Smell is Disease": Miasma, Sensory Rhetoric, and the Sanitary-Bacteriologic of Visceral Public Health," *Rhetoric of Health & Medicine* 2, no. 2 (2019): 115–46.

38 Alaimo, "Trans-corporeal Feminisms and the Ethical Space of Nature," 262.

39 Candice Rai and Gottschalk Drushke, Caroline. *Field Rhetoric: Ethnography, Ecology, and Engagement in the Places of Persuasion* (Tuscaloosa, AL: The University of Alabama Press, 2018), 1.

40 Rai and Gottschalk Drushke, *Field Rhetoric*, 10.

41 Ibid.,16.

42 Ibid., 2.

43 Majno, *The Healing Hand: Man and Wound in the Ancient World*, 170.

44 Ibid., 171.

45 Registered Interpreters for the Deaf. Retrieved from https://rid.org/

46 Anderson, Riker, Gagne, Hakulin, Higgins, Meehan, Stout, Pici-D'Ottavio, Cappetta, and Craig, "Deaf Qualitative Health Research," 1819.

47 Schafer, *The Soundscape*, 7.

48 Thomas R. Lindlof and Bryan C. Taylor, *Qualitative Communication Research Methods* (Sage Publications, 2011), Third edition.

49 Richard A. Lanham, *A Handlist of Rhetorical Terms* (Berkeley, CA: University of California Press, 1991).

50 Lanham, *A Handlist of Rhetorical Terms*, 46.

51 Jennifer Edwell, "Medical Interiors: Materiality and Spatiality in Medical Rhetoric Research Methods," in *Methodologies for the Rhetoric of Health & Medicine*, eds. Lisa Melonçon and J. Blake Scott (New York: Routledge, 2017), 157–75.

52 Lindlof and Taylor, *Qualitative Communication Research Methods*, 89.

53 Bivens, "Rhetorically Listening for Microwithdrawals of Consent in Research Practice."

54 Lindlof and Taylor, *Qualitative Communication Research Methods*, 198.

55 Ibid., 199–202.

56 Bivens, "Rhetorically Listening for Microwithdrawals of Consent in Research Practice," 147.

57 Anderson, Riker, Gagne, Hakulin, Higgins, Meehan, Stout, Pici-D'Ottavio, Cappetta, and Craig, "Deaf Qualitative Health Research," 1817.

58 Registered Interpreters for the Deaf. Retrieved from https://rid.org/

59 Lindlof and Taylor, *Qualitative Communication Research Methods*, 199–202.

60 Anderson, Riker, Gagne, Hakulin, Higgins, Meehan, Stout, Pici-D'Ottavio, Cappetta, and Craig, "Deaf Qualitative Health Research," 1817, 1818.

61 Ibid., 1818.

62 Michel Chion, "The Three Listening Modes," in *The Sound Studies Reader*, ed. Jonathan Sterne (New York: Routledge, 2012), 48.

63 Schafer, *The Soundscape*, 272.

64 Chion, "The Three Listening Modes," 48.

65 Schafer, *The Soundscape*, 272.

66 Ibid., 274.

67 Ibid., 275.

68 Schafer, *The Soundscape*, 274.

69 Lindlof and Taylor, *Qualitative Communication Research Methods*, 278–79.

70 R. Bruce Lindsey, Report to the National Science Foundation on the Conference on Education in Acoustics, *Journal of the Acoustical Society of America* 36 (1964) 2241–44.

71 R. Bruce Lindsey, Erratum: Proceedings of the Conference on Education in Acoustics. *Journal of the Acoustical Society of America*, 37 (1965), 357–81.

72 Schafer, *The Soundscape*, 139–44.

73 Ibid., 141.

74 Schafer, *The Soundscape*, 135.

75 Acoustical Society of America, "Fields of Acoustics." Retrieved from https://exploresound.org/what-is-acoustics/fields-of-acoustics/

76 Bivens, Arduser, Welhausen, and Faris, "A Multisensory Literacy Approach to Biomedical Healthcare Technologies: Aural, Tactile, and Visual Layered Health Literacies," n.p.

77 Eleanor Crossley, Tim Biggs, Phillip Brown, and Tahwinder Singh, "The Accuracy of iPhone Applications to Monitor Environmental Noise Levels," *The Laryngoscope* 131, no. 1 (2021): E59–E62.

78 EA LAB, NIOSH Sound Level Meter. Retrieved from https://apps.apple.com/us/app/niosh-sound-level-meter/id1096545820

79 National Institute for Occupational Safety & Health and EA LAB; Hearing Loss Prevention Team, Engineering and Physical Hazards Branch, Division of Applied Research and Technology. "NIOSH Sound Level Meter." n.d. Retrieved from https://www.cdc.gov/niosh/topics/noise/pdfs/NIOSH-Sound-Level-Meter-Application-app-English.pdf

80 Kathy Charmaz, *Constructing Grounded Theory* (Sage, 2014).

81 Anderson, Riker, Gagne, Hakulin, Higgins, Meehan, Stout, Pici-D'Ottavio, Cappetta, and Craig, "Deaf Qualitative Health Research," 1819.

82 Web Accessibility in Mind, "WebAIM's WCAG 2 Checklist." Retrieved from https://webaim.org/standards/wcag/checklist

83 Lindlof and Taylor, *Qualitative Communication Research Methods*, 155.

84 Ibid., 157.

85 Ibid., 156.

86 Jamie Landau, "Feeling Rhetorical Critics: Another Affective-Emotional Field Method for Rhetorical Studies," *Text+ Field: Innovations in Rhetorical Method* (2016): n.p.

87 Rai and Gottschalk Drushke, *Field Rhetoric*, 4.

88 Web Accessibility in Mind, "WebAIM's WCAG 2 Checklist." Retrieved from https://webaim.org/standards/wcag/checklist

89 Ibid.

90 Florence Nightingale, *Notes on Nursing: What It Is and What It Is Not* (Cambridge: Cambridge University Press, 2010), 67.

91 World Health Organization, Europe, "Noise." 27 April 2010. Retrieved from https://www.who.int/europe/news-room/fact-sheets/item/noise, para. 1.

92 Ibid., para. 2.

93 Birgitta Berglund, Thomas Lindvall, Dietrich H. Schwela, & World Health Organization, Occupational and Environmental Health Team, "Guidelines for community noise," World Health Organization. (1999). Retrieved from https://apps.who.int/iris/handle/10665/66217

94 Abdulraoof Almadhoob, Arne Ohlsson, and Cochrane Neonatal Group, "Sound Reduction Management in the Neonatal Intensive Care Unit for Preterm or Very Low Birth Weight Infants." *Cochrane Database of Systematic Reviews* issue 1 (2020), 1.

95 Sarah J. Sloane, "The Haunting Story of J: Genealogy as a Critical Category in Understanding How a Writer Composes," *Passions, Pedagogies, and 21st century Technologies* (1999): 49–65.

96 Emily S. Rueb, "To Reduce Hospital Noise, Researchers Create Alarms That Whistle and Sing," *The New York Times* (2019), para. 9.

97 Yoko Sen quoted in Rueb, "To Reduce Hospital Noise, Researchers Create Alarms That Whistle and Sing," para. 8.

98 Rueb, "To Reduce Hospital Noise, Researchers Create Alarms That Whistle and Sing," para. 13.

99 Ibid., para. 34.

100 Ibid., para. 42.

101 Ibid., para. 43.

102 McKinnon, Asen, Chávez, and Howard, *Text + Field*, n.p.

103 Ibid.

104 Ceraso, *Sounding Composition*, 112–13.

105 Ibid., 117.

106 Højlund, Marie Koldkjær, "Beyond Insulation and Isolation: Towards an Attuning Approach to Noise in Hospitals," *Sound Effects – An Interdisciplinary Journal of Sound and Sound Experience* 6, no. 1 (2016): 121–40.

107 Ibid., 123.

Index